Operating Room Technique and Anesthesia for General Nursing Course

AF070617

Operating Room Technique and Anesthesia for General Nursing Course

3rd Edition

CP Thresyamma
Rtd Principal (Nursing School)
Perumpallil, Amalagiri PO
Kottayam, Kerala, India

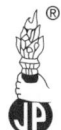

JAYPEE BROTHERS MEDICAL PUBLISHERS (P) LTD
Kochi • St Louis (USA) • Panama City (Panama) • New Delhi • Ahmedabad
Bengaluru • Chennai • Hyderabad • Kolkata • Lucknow • Mumbai • Nagpur

Published by
Jitendar P Vij
Jaypee Brothers Medical Publishers (P) Ltd

Corporate Office
4838/24 Ansari Road, Daryaganj, **New Delhi** - 110002, India
Phone: +91-11-43574357, Fax: +91-11-43574314

Registered Office
B-3 EMCA House, 23/23B Ansari Road, Daryaganj, **New Delhi** - 110 002, India
Phones: +91-11-23272143, +91-11-23272703, +91-11-23282021
+91-11-23245672, Rel: +91-11-32558559, Fax: +91-11-23276490, +91-11-23245683
e-mail: jaypee@jaypeebrothers.com, Website: www.jaypeebrothers.com

Offices in India

- **Ahmedabad**, Phone: Rel: +91-79-32988717, e-mail: ahmedabad@jaypeebrothers.com
- **Bengaluru**, Phone: Rel: +91-80-32714073, e-mail: bangalore@jaypeebrothers.com
- **Chennai**, Phone: Rel: +91-44-32972089, e-mail: chennai@jaypeebrothers.com
- **Hyderabad**, Phone: Rel:+91-40-32940929, e-mail: hyderabad@jaypeebrothers.com
- **Kochi**, Phone: +91-484-2395740, e-mail: kochi@jaypeebrothers.com
- **Kolkata**, Phone: +91-33-22276415, e-mail: kolkata@jaypeebrothers.com
- **Lucknow**, Phone: +91-522-3040554, e-mail: lucknow@jaypeebrothers.com
- **Mumbai**, Phone: Rel: +91-22-32926896, e-mail: mumbai@jaypeebrothers.com
- **Nagpur**, Phone: Rel: +91-712-3245220, e-mail: nagpur@jaypeebrothers.com

Overseas Offices

- **North America Office, USA,** Ph: 001-636-6279734
  e-mail: jaypee@jaypeebrothers.com, anjulav@jaypeebrothers.com
- **Central America Office, Panama City, Panama,** Ph: 001-507-317-0160
  e-mail: cservice@jphmedical.com, Website: www.jphmedical.com

Operating Room Technique and Anesthesia for General Nursing Course

© 2010, CP Thresyamma

All rights reserved. No part of this publication should be reproduced, stored in a retrieval system, or transmitted in any form or by any means: electronic, mechanical, photocopying, recording, or otherwise, without the prior written permission of the author and the publisher.

This book has been published in good faith that the material provided by author is original. Every effort is made to ensure accuracy of material, but the publisher, printer and author will not be held responsible for any inadvertent error(s). In case of any dispute, all legal matters are to be settled under Delhi jurisdiction only.

First Edition : 2002
Second Edition : 2003
Third Edition : **2010**

ISBN 978-81-8448-837-1

Typeset at   JPBMP typesetting unit
Printed at   Rajkamal Electric Press, Plot No. 2, Phase-IV, Kundli, Haryana

Foreword

This book *Operating Room Technique and Anesthesia for General Nursing Course* is an answer to the problem of finding a suitable guide to help the teacher and student alike in the Nursing Education. This book is getting the appreciation of most of the teachers of nursing, both in Nursing School and Hospitals of Private and Public Sectors.

This revised and modified book reflects the knowledge and long experience of the author as a theater nurse and then as a successful teacher in Fundamentals of Nursing. It becomes a superior product when the teacher who knows the disciples and their needs well, gives shape to such a guide that suits to the curriculum. The contents are arranged according to the course outline and the practical record of the student. Matters are presented in very simple language which is an added attraction of this book.

Going through the contents, one can understand that special care has been taken to present it, based on the scientific principles, without sacrificing the practical applicability. This book is a 'must' both for the students, teachers and more so for those nurses who practice in hospitals.

I fervently hope that everyone in the nursing profession will keep a copy of this book and the author will have added spirit to produce more of this kind.

EN Neelakanta Pillai (Late)
Former Nursing Superintendent
MCH Kottayam-1
Kerala, India

Preface to the Third Edition

This book *Operating Room Technique and Anesthesia for General Nursing Course* is prepared according to the method of functioning of the operating rooms in the Medical College Hospitals of Kerala. I think the organization and functioning of operating rooms in Medical College Hospitals of other states will be almost the same although there are slight variations in some matters according to their needs. But the basic principles and practices will be one and the same everywhere.

Operating room is one of the most important departments of the hospital where the people will hesitate to rush in very freely as they enter in other wards of the hospital. There are so many formalities and restrictions to be obliged to enter or work in the operating room for its proper functioning. A nursing student or a new person will have a vague idea about the inside picture of an operating room when compared to the notion about a general ward and that too, might have obtained from the explanation from semiexperienced persons. When a student is posted in the operating room in the first time, she enters there with a wavering mind. Even though there are instructors and supervisors to help her. She is in a dilemma for what to do and what not to do, where to touch and where not to touch, what are the consequences in doing things with anxiety and so on. I am sure that this book will be a good remedy to such uncertainty to some extent.

Theoretical knowledge about disinfection, sterilization, specific functions, performances and responsibilities of each category of people working in the operating room are clearly specified in copious illustrations of needed instruments, their identification and purposes will be very useful in reducing the alarming strangeness of the tools and equipment in the operating room. Selection of the simple language used in the book for presenting the matters will favor the reader to enter the operating room with full confidence.

On the whole, I fully believe that this small book will be a companion and guide to the nursing profession. Also, I am indebted to the appreciations and encouragements received from my co-workers, veteran teachers and other users of this book.

Suggestions for the further improvements will be gratefully accepted.

With best regards.

CP Thresyamma

Preface to the First Edition

Operating Room Technique and Anesthesia for General Nursing Course has been written to better equip the nursing personnel. The students as well as the teachers will find it quite useful.

This revised and modified book reflects the knowledge and long experience of the author as a theatre nurse and then as a teacher in Fundamentals of Nursing. It has been designed in such a manner that it fits in the curriculum. While reading the book the reader will find that the matter has been arranged according to course contents. The presentation is in very simple and lucid language. Special care has been taken to present the matter based on scientific principles without sacrificing the practical applicability.

Analytical comments and suggestions of worthy readers are most welcome for further improvement.

CP Thresyamma

Contents

1. Operating Room: Physical Set-up, OR Team and Functions of Nurses 1
2. Operating Room: Procedure According to the Work Record of the Student 8
3. Operating Table and Positions 13
4. Sterilization and Disinfection 18
5. Common Technical Terms 34
6. Role of the Nurses in Major Operations 42
7. Prevention of Contamination in Operation Room 55
8. Setting up of Instruments 63
9. Instruments: Specifications and their Uses 91
10. Anesthesia 164

    Index *197*

1. Operating Room: Physical Set-up, OR Team and Functions of Nurses

OPERATING ROOM—PHYSICAL SET UP

Operating rooms or the theater block is one of the important special departments of a hospital. An operating room is a particular room where the surgery and the surgical procedures are conducted. This unit is designed as "Self contained block" with a series of rooms leading of a corridor with closed doors that separates it from the general wards but away from the thoroughfare of the hospital. Entrances are provided for bringing and sending patients, instrument trolley, surgical team and other staff members of the unit. Any cross traffics for people other than the workers of the unit are strictly avoided. All the categories of people working in the unit are provided with changing rooms where ordinary cloths can be changed for theater garments or clothing covered with clean gowns, caps and overshoes before entering the operating room or anesthetic rooms. The workers of the unit preserve special foot wear while working hours. This unit is provided with toilet rooms in addition to changing rooms. The surgeons and the sister in charge of the operating room are having their office rooms other than the staff room. Scrubbing room leads directly to the operating room. In some hospitals anesthetic room is separate which opens in to the operating room with serving doors so placed that the patient cannot see the operating room.

Sterilizing equipment is usually placed in an annex leading to the operating room; this arrangement keeps the actual theater free from unnecessary heat and stream and also minimizes noise. These annexes should be large enough to allow sufficient space for the laying up of instruments and other trolleys. A sink room or "utility" room is also necessary in which instruments, bowls, mackintoshes and other equipment can be cleaned after use. A linen room with a large table is a necessity for the sorting and mending of clean linen and for packing drums or making bundles. A stock room may be separated or combined with the linen room.

There should be ample cupboard accommodation. Large or specialized units may include an X-ray room and electric power points are provided in an area accessible to the theater for operating mobile X-ray plants. Separate multiple switch board is of advantage.

Labor-saving and hygienic construction facilitate the daily thorough cleaning which is necessary in all operating rooms. Walls and floors are commonly made with washable materials. The floors should contain "antistatic" material and slope towards a gulley and trapped drain so that the walls and floors can be washed down easily with a hose. As far as possible ledges and corners which may harbor dust are avoided in the construction of the building and in the fittings and furniture. Natural ventilation is seldom possible when a theater is in use, as dust and draughts must be excluded and therefore some form of artificial ventilation is needed. The "plenum" system is frequently used. Air from a reliable source is driven into the theater through filters to remove dirt and impure air is forced out and when necessary the incoming air can be warmed by passing it over heated pipes which can be controlled by the theater staff. If windows are large in order to give plenty of light from outside; blinds are necessary as a protection against too much sunlight in the summer and also to darken the theater when needed for certain operations. The theater needs an efficient system of artificial lighting and an emergency system should be available in the event of the electricity from the main failing. The table lighting is provided by a large shadowless lamp and mobile shadowless "spot lamps". All electric switches in operating theaters and anesthetic rooms should be of the mercury "make and break" type in order to minimize the risk of an explosion caused by sparking.

Theater furnishings and fittings should be made of stainless steel for quick and thorough cleaning. Trolleys of all types should be fitted with large casters made up of conducting rubber to minimize sparking from static electricity. The modern operating rooms are air conditioned and the walls and furnishings are of pleasing colors or white.

Special laundry facilities should be provided in the operating unit. This arrangement not only prevents the delay of getting fresh clean linen but also exclude the chance of mixing the linen with linen of other departments of the hospital. It also prolongs the duration of the use of the same linen, prevents much damage and loss and reduces the chances of infection. In short, operating room block is a *self contained unit* of the hospital pertaining to the staff and functioning. *The operating room technique* describe the methods of routine functioning of this unit.

Several operating rooms are seen in one unit because the special operations other than general surgery are done in their own rooms such as neurosurgery, orthopedic surgery, ENT operations, eye operations, paediatric surgery, thoracic surgery, gynecologic surgery, etc. Surgeons and nurses working in each room will be specialized in that branch of surgery. The nurse who is specialized in the operating room technique and the one who is the seniormost of them will be in charge of the unit. She controls the functioning of the operating room team work and the anesthetic section.

THE CATEGORIES OF PEOPLE IN THE OPERATING ROOM TEAM WORK

Surgeons: Specialized in the particular branch of surgery.

Assistant surgeons: Specialized but practising with the senior surgeon.

House surgeons: If it is medical college hospital.

Medical students: If any.

Theater sister: Seniormost and specialized in OR techniques.

Other theater nurses: Specialized to work in special operating rooms.
- Head nurses
- Staff nurses
- 2nd and 3rd year nursing students.
- Operating room technicians.
- Other workers such as attenders, cleaners, *dobhi*, etc.
- The number of nurses and other workers depends upon the type of hospital and the number of daily operations.
- Anesthetic section functions in the equal level along with surgical team under the chief anesthetist. They include:
  - Chief anesthetist (doctor)
  - Other assistant anesthetist (doctors)
  - House surgeons and medical students, if any
  - Anesthetist nurse who is specialized in anesthesia
  - Other staff nurses and nursing students (2nd and 3rd years)
  - One or two attenders.
- Here also, type and number of staff members depends upon the number of daily operations.

Surgical team and anesthetic team function inseparable and the sister in charge of the operating room looks after the welfare of both sections.

GENERAL FUNCTIONS OF OPERATING ROOM NURSES

The theater nurse should aim at attaining an efficient standard of aseptic technique and such a well developed surgical conscience that she can be relied upon to carry out her work at all times and particularly under conditions of emergency, with speed, accuracy, and calmness. Such a desirable standard is not obtained without a thorough knowledge of the principles of sterilization and theater technique. Every nurse working in the theater needs to realize that the success of the surgeon's work depends largely on the careful reliable attention in detail shown by every member of the staff and the keenness, sharp observation, and dexterity which will make each member of the theater personnel an efficient unit, in the surgical team.

In the theaters, nurses usually change into white shortsleeved dresses of over all type, theater caps covering the hair, masks, white shoes and stockings before beginning the preparation of instruments, apparatus, and lotions for the day's operations. Ward nurses, students and visitors when entering in the theater are also required to change or to cover their ordinary clothing with clean gowns, to wear caps and masks and to put on white rubber or canvas boots over their shoes.

Theater linen is used for patient's trolleys. Only the minimum of ward linen, e.g. the patients gown, should be brought to the theater and must always be freshly laundered. These precautions are necessary in order to reduce the risk of wound infection.

During operations: The sister or nurse who is to act as the "instrument nurse" scrubs up, covers her theater dress with a sterilized gown, and puts on sterilized rubber gloves.

The instrument nurse checks and arranges the instruments on the instrument table and passes them to the surgeon, as far as possible anticipating his needs. She also prepares ligatures and sutures, having them ready for the different stages of the operation. She passes mops and gauze pads to the surgeon and his assistant, is responsible for accounting for all swabs and instruments, including needles at any stage of the operation and in particular before any cavity is closed. During all bone operations, and for some surgeons during any type of operation, all instruments, swabs, all ligatures and sutures may be handled with forceps so that no sterile materials coming in contact with the wound, is touched by the gloved hands.

One, or if possible, two nurses who will not scrub up will act as runners or 'circulating' nurses. One of these should watch the instrument nurse and be ready to bring anything that she may require or to put any extra instruments in the sterilizers as directed. It will be one of the duties to keep the sterilizers filled with water and boiling and to see that the instruments are ready for the next case. She assists in placing the patient on the theater table if a theater porter is not available.

The second runner hand over gowns, caps and gloves to the surgeon and assistants, removing these articles from the drums with long handled forceps. She also ties the gowns. She puts the lotions in the lotion bowls and changes them as necessary. For some operations hot sterile normal saline solution is required. She replenishes the mops and pads as they are used and is responsible for checking the used swaps and displaying them on the counting stand. If a tourniquet is applied to a patient in the theater the time at which it is to be removed should be written down and subsequently entered in the patient's history sheet. When the other runner is in the sterilizing room she must watch the instrument nurse and be ready to attend to any needs. At no time during the operation should the theater be left without one runner.

The ward nurse in charge of the patient should see that all records such as case notes and X-ray films (with the consent to operation form uppermost) are brought to the theater with the patient. She should be able to answer questions concerning the preparation of the patient, e.g. when the premedication was given or when the patient had his last feed. She remains with her patient in the anesthetic room until the patient is unconscious. Then, with the anesthetist's permission she returns to the ward. If the local anesthesia or no anesthesia is planned, she will put on theater clothing and accompany the patient into the theatre. In some cases the entire preparation of the skin, beginning with shaving and cleaning with ether, may be undertaken in the theatre. Usually the final preparation only is carried out on the operating table. This may consists of vigorous sponging of the area with a gauze mop soaked in cetrimide and held with sponge forceps. This is followed by mopping with a dry swab and finally painting the area with surgical spirit or with an antiseptic such a s 2.5 percent iodine in spirit or Hibitane 0.5 percent in 70 percent alcohol. The ward nurse is responsible for taking any instructions regarding the care of the patient, from the surgeon or anesthetist, back to the ward sister.

Most theaters keep a daily register of operations in which the nature of the operation, its duration and the anesthetic used are entered up for each case. The book is usually signed by the instrument nurse and by the anesthetist. Another operation register is maintained for the surgeon with the details of operations for each unit.

Modern concept is that the energy and time of a qualified nurse is not wasted to work as a circulating nurse. But they can be improvised by competent technicians. Also the working personnel in the OR unit is not interchangeable from a ward to theater or from the theater to wards for temporary adjustments as practised in general wards.

The set up and functioning of the operating room is aimed at the maintenance of the aseptic condition of the unit, the successful surgery and an uneventful postoperative period of every patient.

2. Operating Room: Procedure According to the Work Record of the Student

PREPARATION OF ANESTHETIC TABLE

Many patients are naturally apprehensive from the time they enter into the operating room until they are anesthetized. So it is better to have the anesthetic room separate, provided with a door leading to the operating room so that the patient is anesthetized before he is taken to the operation room. In many hospitals the patient is anesthetized in the operation table itself. In both the conditions all the preparations are carried out before the arrival of the patient.

The premedication, according to the type of anesthesia is given sufficiently early. Anesthetic trolley, Boyle's machine, spinal anesthesia trolley and the tray for the local anesthesia should be prepared ready before hand. A suction apparatus is essential especially in general anesthesia.

Anesthesia trolley contains all the accessories for giving anesthesia, drugs required for the whole day depending upon the number of cases to be operated. Every day morning, the things are removed from the trolley and the trolley is cleaned by wet wiping and disinfected with carbolic lotion. Medicine trays are replenished. Sufficient number and types of syringes are kept sterile on the trolley.

Oxygen cylinders and other cylinders for gases are replenished with full cylinders every morning. They should be checked for good working conditions for immediate use. Rubber catheters, rubber tubes and glass connections should be kept ready on the trolley for the convenient use of the anesthetist.

Boyle's apparatus and suction apparatus should be checked for good working condition before hand. Usually the anesthetists prefer to start the intravenous infusion to the patient after anesthesia is induced but before operation. So, articles and solutions required for the IV infusion should be ready near the anesthetic trolley. (More details are learned from the notes of anesthesia).

PREPARATION OF THEATER AND EQUIPMENT

Operation room is a place where absolute cleanliness should be maintained. Minimize the equipment as far as possible. The articles required are operation table, the trolleys required for setting instruments: stands for keeping lotion and a wall board for writing the number of mops and the materials mentioned for anesthesia. All these furniture and fittings should be wiped with duster dipped and squeezed in disinfectant lotion everyday morning. Carbolizing is done after wet-wiping. Dry dusting is avoided always. Floor and walls are as important as the other furniture in the room. Nail brushes are sterilized either by boiling or autoclaving and kept in sterile containers in the sink room. Separate soap pieces are kept at each sink near the sterile brush container. In case a septic condition is dealt in the theater, the whole place including the operation table along with all the other articles require a thorough washing with soap and water followed by an antiseptic lotion, before arranging any other operation.

All the people working in the theater, use special dresses and shoes which are kept only for the time of theater work. Anyone entering inside the theater after carbolising should wear cap and mask along with the theater gown.

SETTING UP OF STERILE TROLLEY

The theater nurse after scrubbing, puts sterile cap, mask, gown and gloves. The running nurse opens the sterile drum and handles the sterile towel with a transfer forceps to the sterile nurse. The towel should be sufficiently large enough to spread on the trolley covering its sides. The instrument nurse spreads the towel very carefully on the trolley without making the part on the trolley unsterile and without touching her gloved hands on any unsterile area.

The sterile nurse takes the instruments, drapings and all the other sterile items required, from the sterile drum or packet as the case may be, which is opened by the runner and arrange it neatly on the trolley according to the order of use. She counts the number of mops and arrange to mark it on the board before starting the operation. After arranging, the trolley is covered by a sterile towel till it is handed over to the surgeon as required or spread in the tray adjusted over the operation table at the foot end.

SCRUBBING

Hands cannot be rendered sterile by scrubbing with soap, water and brush. As dirt is a potential source of infection, all dirt must be removed from the hands before operation. Dirt is present on the surface of the hands, forearms, in the creases of the skin, beneath the nail folds and around the base of the nail. All the nurses working in the theater must observe certain rules about the cleanliness of their hands.

1. During the period of theater work, hands should not be allowed to come in contact with pus or infected dressings. Forceps should be used in all such occasions.
2. Avoid injury to the hands as far as possible. Nail polish should not be used during theater work.
3. Nails should be kept short so that dirt do not gather beneath them and keep the hands always as clean as possible.

Before scrubbing, hands should be washed with soap and water for one minute to remove the superficial dirt. Then the cap and mask provided are put on. After that the hands are scrubbed for 5 (five) minutes seeing a clock, with soap, sterile nail brush and running water. Special attention is required in the method of scrubbing. Fingers and hands should be extended to open the creases of the skin. Care should be taken not to neglect the webs of the fingers, ball of the thumb and the nail folds which are the places often inadequately cleaned. This scrubbing extends upto elbows and in two sessions.

That is first one and a half minute is used for scrubbing: half a minute for washing which is one session.

Second session of scrubbing lasts for two minutes and washing for the last one minute. Total 5 minutes.

For final washing care should be taken not to allow the water to run from the arm to the palm. Hold the palms together pointing fingers up so that water will flow from palms to around the elbow. Also, in between scrubbing by the small piece of soap and nail brush, it should be changed in hands; from right to left and left to right hands as required. Once we have taken the soap and brush in hand for scrubbing it should not be put down till the scrubbing is finished after five minutes. It is very effective if we use ether soap for washing the hands after scrubbing and washing with brush, soap and water.

Preparation of Ether Soap

Make a thick jelly of carbolic soap and water by melting the soap on heater or stove in a basin. Cool it well. Add ether sufficient to make the thick jelly to be diluted so that it can be poured to a bottle and from the bottle back for use. Keep it in an air tight bottle in the scrubbing room. This can be used instead of soap for scrubbing as well as for washing hands after scrubbing. It is a very good detergent.

Five minutes of intelligent scrubbing of this type is much more effective than a longer period of purposeless scrubbing. After five minutes, wash off the soap well and dry the hand with a sterile towel. Use spirit for further drying.

Theater sinks are provided with taps which can be manipulated with upper arm or foot operated, so that we should not close the tap with hands after washing. Once the hands have been scrubbed and dried, it should be held away from the body and at a higher level than the elbows.

Nurses who have to scrub their hands frequently should be very careful to use good nail brush and not to make their hands raw because bacteria from deep in the skin come to the surface and are difficult to remove owing to the soreness of the skin. It is better if they use a soft hand cream for the care of sensitive skin.

The time and sessions of scrubbing with plenty of soap lather and nail brush vary in hospitals and persons within the time of five minutes. Still the effect required and the principles are same everywhere. Some other non-irritating skin cleansing agents such as ether soap or other readymade preparations also are good. Between cases, after discarding the gloves the hands are well washed with soap lather and scrubbing for 3 minutes and drying with sterile towel is also practiced. There are different opinion about the time of scrubbing among surgeons and in different hospitals. In some books it is said as 5 minutes whereas in some other books, it is said as 5 to 10 minutes. But some surgeons used to scrub for 15 minutes whereas some others take even less than 5 minutes:

The duration of the scrub may be determined by a time limit set on the conscientious scrubbing of one part after another in a prescribed manner or it may be determined by a certain number of strokes per part. A practical, reliable and intelligent procedure should be practiced. It is better to set up a standard time in each hospital by a committee on aseptic procedure.

GOWNING

The scrubbing nurse handles the sterile gown very carefully without touching on her body and slips into its sleeves gently over her theater dress. The gown is tied by the "runner" (Demonstration), at the back. The hands at the wrist are tied by herself so that the cuffs of the gloves are fitted over them.

GLOVING

The sterile packets are opened carefully. One glove has been put on with the cuff still turned back. She puts the second glove with the gloved hand touching only the outside of the second glove. Complete the process by pulling the cuffs of the gloves over the sleeves of the sterile gown at the wrist (Demonstration).

3

Operating Table and Positions

OPERATING TABLE

The modern operating table is designed to facilitate various positioning for the different operations. It has got several fittings, which are easily operatable even during the process of surgery. The theater nurse should be quite familiar with the working of the particular table so that she can make any desired adjustments speedily before and during the progress of operation. Extra table fittings should never be placed on the floor. But it should be kept on a side trolley for the easy supply at any time when required. The operating table consists of three pieces for easy adjustments; a small head piece, big middle piece for the trunk and a lower piece for the lower extremity. An adjustable kidney bridge is fitted on the middle piece of the table at the kidney level of an adult patient.

The positioning of the table should be done very carefully that there should not be any harm to the patient from pressure especially on nerves. Making any change in the position of the patient during operation must be done only with the permission of the anesthetist. Great care must be taken to prevent any injury to the arms when moving an unconscious patient. If one arm is underneath the body, it should either be supported in the natural position of flexion or straightened. On the table the patient should be carefully placed especially when he is unconscious. Infants may be bandaged to a well padded cruciform splint. *Never leave a patient alone on the table before, during or after operation,* irrespective of whether he is conscious or unconscious because the table is less wide and he may fall down on moving himself.

SOME OF THE SPECIAL POSITIONING OF THE OPERATING TABLE

Laparotomy Position

The patient is placed supine with the arms at the sides and the hands pronated with the thumbs underneath the body. The table is adjusted to the height convenient for the surgeon.

Nephrectomy or Kidney Position

The patient is placed in the lateral position with the affected side uppermost. The underneath leg is fully flexed at the knee with the foot placed under the upper leg. Pads are used to prevent skin friction. The bridge of the table is raised to elevate the loin region between the lower ribs and iliac crest. The uppermost arm is supported on a padded rest and the underneath arm is pulled a little away from the body and flexed at the elbow with the hand under the patient's face.

This position, but usually without the raised bridge, is used for rib resection, for draining an empyema and also for thoracoplasty.

Lithotomy Position

The position receives its name from the fact that it was used for one of the commonest operations of the past; lithotomy or cutting the bladder for the removal of stone, It is used for operations on the perineum, anal region and external genital organs.

The patient is placed on the table so that the buttocks project well over the junction of the middle and lower sections of the table. The end of the table is then lowered to the vertical position. The patient's legs are raised and flexed at the hips and knees with the feet supported in the webbing slings of the crutches fixed to the sides of the table. Two persons are required to raise the patient's legs at the same time in order to avoid the danger of a fracture as for example in the case of a patient with arthritis of the hip joint.

Small pads are used to prevent pressure of the metal poles on the patient's thighs. The patient's hands are placed on her chest.

Many gynecologists and urological surgeons now prefer modified lithotomy position in which the thighs are less acutely flexed and the legs are supported by leg rests in place of the stirrups and poles.

Cholecystectomy or Gallbladder Position

The patient is supine with the arms extended on padded support. The bridge of the table is raised under the lower ribs in order to push the liver and gallbladder forward against the anterior abdominal wall. The break of the table can be used instead of a bridge.

The arms are never fixed at the side for this operation but should be either extended on arm boards or flexed across the upper chest and fixed with wide strapping.

The bridge is lowered or the break straightened before closure of the peritoneum.

Trendelenburg Position

The patient is placed supine so that the bend of the knees is exactly over the junction of the foot and central section of the table. The foot end of the table is slightly lowered so that the patient's knees are flexed slightly.

Pelvic supports to retain the patient in this position are now commonly used in place of shoulder rests in order to avoid the danger of paralysis of the arms from pressure on the nerves of the brachial plexus. The head end of the table is slightly lower than the foot end by tilting it.

The object of the Trendelenburg position is to allow the intestines to fall away from the pelvic cavity towards the upper abdomen.

Positions for Operations on the Breast and Axilla

The patient is placed supine with the arms extended on a padded rest. A small pillow may be placed under the chest and axilla on the affected side. An alternative position is to bring the arm away from the body by flexing it at the elbow and tying it by a clove hitch round the wrist above the patient's head to the stand of the instrument tray at the head of the table. The arm may also be held in this position by an assistant seated on a stool at the head end of the table.

Position for Operations in the Neck

This is the position used for thyroidectomy and for tracheostomy.

The patient is placed supine with one or two sand bags under the shoulders so that the head is hyperextended. The anesthetist steadies the patient's head.

The sand bag is removed to allow a position of slight flexion before suturing begins. Great care is needed to support the head in a position of slight flexion in all postoperative movement of the patient in order to preserve the sutures intact in the platysma-muscle. This position with slight alteration used for tonsillectomy is called Rose's position.

Position for Cerebellar Operations and High Laminectomy

The patient's eyes in the prone position and is moved up the table so that the head projects over the end and is supported by the forehead resting in the horseshoe which is fixed about 6 inches (15 cm) below the level of the table top. A small pillow or rubber wedge is placed under the upper part of the chest. The patient's arms lie at the sides with thumbs just under the thighs.

The patient's eyes should be protected by a dressing fixed with adhesive strapping or eye pad. The anesthetic tubing should also be secured.

A small pillow under the pelvis prevents pressure on the abdominal aorta and pads under the lower parts of the leg allow a normal position for the feet.

Laminectomy in the thoracic and lumbar regions is sometimes performed with the patient in the lateral position. The knees should be fully flexed and fixed in this position with adhesive strapping. The strapping is released when the surgeon begins the suturing of the wound. Sandbags and a pelvic post support the trunk on the ventral aspect. The upper arm may be supported on an arm rest.

Position for Bronchoscopy and Esophagoscopy

A special table may be used or an adjustable head rest clamped to the end of the ordinary theater table. The patient's shoulders are brought to the upper edge of the table and head supported in the rest. The wheel seen on the right hand side of the table alters the position of the rest so that the patient's head can be raised or lowered as desired. The triple sheath above the wheel, which is detachable for sterilization holds the bronchoscope or esophagoscope and suction tubes. The padded clamps just below the shoulders help to steady the patient.

4 Sterilization and Disinfection

STERILIZATION

Complete destruction of micro-organisms is called sterilization. A material is said to be sterile when it is free from all micro-organisms. There is no midway between sterile and unsterile. Complete sterilization of instrument and equipment is used in the surgical practice. It is effected by exposure to high temperature for sufficient length of time to kill all living organisms and their spores. Heat is the most efficient agent whenever its use is possible in the form of high pressure steam sterilizers (autoclaves). Hot air ovens and boiling water sterilizers are also in common use and with proper care and precautions, it can be regarded as reasonably safe for the sterilization of metal equipment such as instruments and bowls.

Disinfection by chemical agents is used for materials and equipment which cannot stand exposure to heat such as endoscopes, bronchoscopes, etc. Chemical disinfectants are also used for disinfection of the skin and the irrigation of body cavities.

All methods of sterilization begin with thorough cleansing of the equipment. Cleanliness is the basis of sterilization. So irrespective of the method of sterilization and disinfection, the materials should be absolutely clean.

Sterilization by Heat

1. Autoclaving (moist heat) or steam under pressure.
2. Dry heat.
3. Boiling.

Autoclaving

Since moist heat is the most effective means of sterilization, it is used whenever possible. Steam under pressure which is an autoclave is recognized as the best method of sterilization where the material will stand this treatment. Steam kills organisms by coagulations of the cell protein; provided that certain factors are present; the steam must be under pressure, dry and saturated. With these conditions fulfilled, the steam will condense when it meets the cooler surface of the article in the autoclave and the latent heat released on condensation will penetrate and kill the organisms. Autoclaving at a pressure of 20 Ibs per square inch and a temperature of 126°C (260°F) for twenty minutes is an efficient method of sterilizing fabrics such as gowns, towels and dressings and also instruments. The latest type of high speed, high vacuum autoclaves operating at higher temperatures reduce the time needed for sterilization. Rubber is readily damaged by exposure to high temperatures for long periods, such as are necessitated during the process of creating a vacuum and subsequent drying process in all but the most modern autoclaves. Rubber gloves are usually autoclaved at a lower temperature, e.g. 121°C (250°F), for ten minutes. The gloves should be very loosely packed, in order to ensure full penetration of the steam.

It is important to remember that any sterilization by autoclaving is reliable only if the autoclave is correctly installed, efficiently operated and the materials packed loosely so that all parts are accessible to the steam. The operation of the autoclave is a serious responsibility and should be entrusted only to one who understands its working. Tests of efficiency, in addition to checking the accuracy of the pressure gauges and temperature readings, should be carried out at regular intervals; these include indicators, control tubes and bacteriological tests.

Signaloc

Signaloc is an autoclave table to check the sterilization of materials, 2.5 × 10 cm, tapes are available in cardboard packets. If the sterilization is cent percent, color change is indicated on the tabel.

So before keeping the things inside the autoclave, a strip of signaloc is pasted on the packet. Lengthwise half of the tape is slightly green originally which is pasted on the packet. If the sterilization is perfect, green color change into dark black in color. If no color change, it means sterilization is not complete and autoclave is not working properly.

Dry Heat

Dry heat kills micro-organisms by oxidation provided that the articles to be sterilized are exposed to a temperature of 160°C (320°F) for one hour, all organisms and their spores will be destroyed. This method is suitable for all types of glass ware including glass syringe (but not glass and metal syringes where the solder will melt in high temperature in the oven) and some instruments such as knife, blades and skin-grafting knives.

Boiling

All pathogenic organisms in the vegetative form and many spore forms are killed by five minutes immersion in boiling water, although there are resistant spores which will withstand long periods of boiling. If the water is made alkaline its lethal effect is increased: therefore sodium carbonate is added to the water in which instruments are boiled if this method of preparation is used. 2% solution of sodium carbonate also retards rusting and reduces the blunting of sharp instruments during boiling. In order that this method of sterilization may be as efficient as possible the following points should be carefully observed.
1. The water must be boiling for the full five minutes. The addition of a large number of cold metal instruments to the water reduce the boiling point.
   The water must be boiling again before the five minutes time is begun.
2. All instruments in the sterilizer must be completely immersed in the water.
3. After use all instruments must be boiled for five minutes and carefully dried before being put away.

4. Instruments when not in use must be stored in a dustfree and dust proof instrument cupboard.
5. The material to be sterilized must be either a good conductor of heart, such as metal, or so constructed that all surfaces are easily reached by the boiling water. Material such as thread wound on reels requires a longer period of boiling because the heat does not penetrate at once to the inner layers.

In cases where contamination with spore-forming organisms, such as anthrax or tetanus organisms are suspected, all instruments and other articles which have been used should either be autoclaved or subjected to prolonged and repeated boiling. The articles should first be boiled for one hour and after a period allowed for cooling: the boiling should be repeated for a further hour. Any spores which have escaped destruction will revert to the vegetative form during the interval and are then killed during the second boiling. This method is called *intermittent sterilization*.

Disinfection by Chemicals

These methods must be used only for the preparation of non-boilable surfaces. Disinfection by chemicals is effective if and only if, the articles are thoroughly cleaned and free of debris, blood, pus, oil and grease. The presence of organic matter greatly diminish the efficiency of the chemical and in some cases may inhibit its action altogether. Oil and grease may be removed by washing the articles in a detergent agent such as 1 percent cetrimide. Penetration of the chemical into the joint of the scissors and forceps may be slow and this sort of immersion will be effective only if the disinfectant solution has rapid access to all surfaces. Whenever, possible instruments should be taken to pieces for chemical sterilization. Antiseptic solutions are also used in the preparation of the patient's skin for operation and for the irrigation of body cavities.

Preparation and Sterilization

1. *Rubber Goods*

Rubber tubing, drainage tubes, rubber catheters and tracheal tubes are sterilized by boiling for five minutes or by autoclaving. Care should be taken to keep the material immersed during boiling and it is necessary to expel air bubbles first and in some cases to weigh the rubber articles in order to keep them immersed. Put a piece of wet cotton over the rubber tube so that the weight of the wet cotton will keep the tube immersed under water while boiling.

After use careful washing is necessary, especially if the tubing is stained with blood, as these stains are difficult or impossible to remove after boiling. The lumen of tubing is best cleaned by attaching the tubing to a pressure nozzle of a cold water supply and forcing water through it. In the case of suction tubing, this must be done very thoroughly. Rolling the tubing under the hand on a board will help to loosen any particles adhering to the interior of the tubing. The tubing is then well washed in warm soapy water, rinsed, boiled for five minutes and hung up to dry. Rubber catheters are cleaned in the same way. Passing of stillet or thin wire through the lumen of the rubber tube or catheters is of great use to clean the inside and to remove block.

The rubber face pieces of the anesthetic apparatus and rubber airway are washed in warm, soapy water after use and boiled for five minutes. The spigot in the cushion must be removed before the face piece is boiled. Chemical disinfectants should not be used because instances have occurred of irritation of the skin of the patients face due to the chemical absorbed by the rubber during immersion.

2. Gloves

Rubber gloves are sterilized by autoclaving at a pressure of 15 lbs, for ten minutes. Talcum powder which was once widely used as a glove powder, is replaced by a prepared corn starch powder. It has been found that grains of talc: implanted in operation wounds from gloves or mackintoshes can produce granulomatous reactions leading to the formation of adhesions. Corn starch produces no such action and the mixture of amylase and amylopectin obtained from this source treated to prevent gelatinization, is obtainable under the name of Biosorb powder or K.285 prepared corn starch powder. It can be sterilized by autoclaving and is preferably packed with the gloves in small paper envelopes.

When gloves are removed after use they may be discarded into a pail containing soapy water. At the end of the operation, used gloves are removed from the pail, washed in warm soapy water, rinsed well and tested for holes. The gloves are then hung up to dry, keeping intact gloves separate from those with holes. When dry on the outside they are turned and left until both surfaces are dry. Undamaged gloves are grouped in sizes and put away. Patched gloves are not suitable for theater use but may be used in wards and departments for examination purposes or for barrier nursing.

3. *Gum Elastic and Plastic Materials*

Some of these materials can be autoclaved or boiled and the instructions given by the manufacturers should be followed. If the material cannot be subjected to heat without risk of damage, the articles should be immersed in bactericidal solution such as 2 percent solution of chlorhexidine (Hibitane) or 1 percent domiphen bromide (Bradosol) solution for twenty minutes. Phenol disinfectants must not be used for elastic gum or plastic materials, as these articles will be damaged by phenol.

Hollow instruments such as catheters if treated by chemical disinfection should be filled with the solution and immersed in a vertical tank in order to get rid of air bubbles.

4. *Surgical Dressings and Linen Drapes*

All types of cotton materials such as gauze, cotton wool and bandages are autoclaved in drums. Dressings for use in the theater are usually larger in size than those commonly used for ward dressings. Swabs and dressing materials such as gauze, cotton wool and cellulose can now be obtained ready. Made, prepared in a great variety of shapes and sizes. Dressings must be packed loosely in drums or packets to be sterilized by autoclaving.

Small and large swabs and pads used during operations may be made of gauze or muslin. The size required will depend on the type of operation and the choice of the surgeon. Small mops may be made up in the packets of ten lightly bundled together to facilitate counting. The bundles should be checked by a second person before they are packed for sterilization. Large pads, sometimes known as abdominal or laparotomy pads, are made of thirty-two layers of gauze about 9 inches by 14 inches. The layers are stitched together with a sewing machine so that there are no loose threads and a tape is sewn to one corner. Some surgeons use swabs with a metal thread running through the gauze, should there be any question of a swab having been left in the abdominal or any other cavity the metal thread will show in an X-ray film; alternatively a fine plastic tube loaded with barium, which is opaque to X-rays may be incorporated in the swabs. It should be remembered that such specially prepared swabs are more expensive than plain gauze and therefore they should not be used as ordinary dressing material for covering a wound. Loose mops can be used for superficial operations where there is no chance of a swab being overlooked. In some theaters loose mops are colored, for example, green and counted mops are left white.

Gauze rolls 3 yards long and 6 inch wide made by folding 12 inches into three and rolled are used for packing off a part or a cavity, e.g. during a gallbladder operation or partial gastrectomy, and may also be used for dressing as for example, on an amputation stump.

One inch ribbon gauze is used for small mops for operations on the lung, in neurosurgery, for thyroid operations and in lengths for nose and ear surgery.

Small lintin or gauze swabs are useful in neurosurgery; these have a black silk thread attached.

Lintin is a wood-pulp dressing which can be cut into strips which are soft and have no loose threads. This is a useful mopping material, particularly in small cavities.

Wool rolls, cellulose, and gamgee may be used for outer dressings and packing. Roller bandages in varying widths from 1 to 6 inches are required sterile for some operations on the limbs.

Eye dressings: The eye drum is packed with small mops of best quality gauze, eye pads of gamgee or best quality cotton wool and eye bandages. The latter are made from a piece of cotton material, preferably a fine quality 6 inches long and 2 inches wide, with a small notch cut in the lower border to accommodate the nose. A tape about 4 inches long is sewn on each of the four corners. At each side, the ends of the two tapes are sewn together and at the joint a single tape is attached which is long enough to pass round the back of the head and round to front again where the two tapes are tied in a bow over a wool mop. To cover the face, square muslin with holes cut for the eyes, can be used in place of a sterile towel. Oiled silk is used in certain dressing, e.g. colostomy.

Cotton drapes such as sheets and towels and gowns must be inspected to ensure that they are clean and free from holes before being packed for sterilizing. They should be folded in such a way that they can be handled when required by a sterile assistant (or by unsterile assistant using cheatle's forceps) maintaining a sterile surface. Rubber sheeting should be folded with a cotton sheet to aid penetration of steam and also subsequent drying. All these articles must be loosely packed for autoclaving. The size and types of drapings and the number of drapings varies in various theaters depending upon the routine of the hospital or the interest of individual surgeons. Sterilizing period is 20 minutes at a pressure of 20 lbs with a temperature of 260°F.

The holes in the sides of the drum should be positively opened before putting them in the autoclave. As soon as the drum is taken from the autoclave after sterilization these holes must be closed. Then only the quality of sterilization retains. The pattern of bundles in special cotton bags also is followed in some hospitals instead of packing in drums. The packets are taken only in sterile trays to field of use for handling to the instrument nurse.

5. *Sterile Water and Infusion Fluids*

The bottle should not be full with solution for autoclaving. There should be an allowance of space in the bottle to permit the expansion of fluid when heated. Solutions should not be autoclaved along with any other articles. The mouths of the bottles should be covered with several thickness of gauze or one layer of lint tightened with a string at its neck or very loosely covered with its own screw cap. As soon as it is taken away from the autoclave after sterilization and became cold, bottles should be tightly screwed and preserved in almarrha. The time and amount of temperature are same as that of surgical dressing. Bottles of water and saline solution are sterilized by autoclaving in screw-capped bottles. Unless very special precautions are taken, any bottles of sterile water or sterile saline solution, should be regarded as contaminated once it has been opened. Unless the seal is unbroken, the contents of the bottle should not be used for rinsing instruments removed from disinfectants or for washing instruments during operations. Once the screw cap has been removed and the contents exposed to the air the label "sterile" on the bottle is meaningless. Screw cap should be used in preference to stoppers as they protect the rim of the bottle from contamination.

6. **Instruments**

Metal instruments are two types boilable and nonboilable. Boilable instruments are packed separate. This packings are usually done as a particular set of instruments required for the particular operation which is the common practice for the planned operations. Several sets of instruments are preserved for meeting the emergency operations to use at any time depending upon the usual occurrence of emergencies in the particular hospital. Sharp instruments as blade and scissors are covered in a piece of lint or gauze to prevent rubbing their sharp edges with other instruments and thereby reducing their sharpness.

Nonboilable instruments may be of different groups such as cystoscopes, bronchoscopes, etc. with special electric fittings of bulb and wires which may be spoiled by boiling. Such materials are sterilized or disinfected by chemical agents.

The sterilization of boilable and nonboilable instruments are given separate.

Boilable Instruments

The time and temperature required are same as that of surgical dressings. Metal instruments, including scissors and needles, are either boiled or autoclaved. Detachable knife blades and scalpels may also be autoclaved or sterilized by dry heat.

The care and cleaning of instruments is an important duty. *After use all sharp instruments and needles are separated from the group.* Then all instruments should be thoroughly scrubbed with a fairly stiff brush under running cold water and then boiled for five minutes. They are taken out of the sterilizer and thoroughly dried while still hot. They should then be examined and oiled as necessary with a fine machine oil, with particular attention paid to the joints of such instruments as forceps and scissors. If oil is used, it is removed before sterilization. Any instruments needing repair or resharpening are then put aside. Sharp instruments must be handled with the greatest care, particularly delicate knives such as cataract knives should never be picked up by the blade. Scissors need only occasional sharpening if they are of good quality.

Nonboilable instruments: Some instruments need special care and it is important to follow meticulously the directions given by the makers. It is difficult to give exact rules for the sterilization of all types of endoscopes (i.e. electrically illuminated instruments for the examination of various body cavities and passages such as cystoscopes, sigmoidoscopes, bronchoscopes and esophagoscopes), but the makers usually specify which parts of the instrument cannot be subjected to heat in the case of the "nonboilable" types. Those instruments which are made to withstand the boiling of all parts must be warmed and boiled gradually as they may be damaged if suddenly plunged into boiling water. Sudden cooling by immersion in cold water after boiling may also damage optical instruments. In the Nonboilable type, the telescope, light and light carriers are immersed in phenylmercuric nitrate or (acetate) solution 1 in 10,000 and other parts of the instrument can be boiled.

Leads from the electric supply to endoscopes or to diathermy apparatus can usually be boiled for five minutes in water without the addition of soda. If they cannot be boiled, formalin vapor is the most suitable method of sterilization. Diathermy electrodes if not boilable are sterilized either in formalin vapor or in phenylmercuric acetate solution. Bronchoscopes, laryngoscopes and esophagoscopes are often kept in a formalin cabinet and are considered to be sterile after twelve hours in the vapor.

After use, endoscopes should be washed in cetrimide, the boilable parts are boiled and nonboilable parts are placed in one of the disinfectant solutions mentioned above for twenty minutes. A fine brush should be used to clean the interior of sheaths. The apparatus is then dried. Alcohol can be used to dry the interior of the hollow parts but must not come in contact with the cement of the lenses. When the instruments are reassembled, valves lights and leads should all be tested.

7. *Suture Needles*

Needles may be fixed on a piece of lint to prevent missing among instruments and boiled or autoclaved along with the other instruments. Usually needles required for a particular operations are sterilized along with their own set of instruments.

In some hospitals the sterilization of needles and sharp instruments are done by the use of chemical agents. Then the time and strength of the lotion required for sterilization depends upon the type of agent used for it.

More Details about Needles

Suture needles may be classified according to the:
1. Thickness and size
2. Curve
3. Use

1. *Thickness and Size*

Needles may be very small, medium size and large.
a. Very small needles, e.g. VVF needles, eye needles, etc.
b. Medium size: Cervix needles, intestinal needles, etc.
c. Large size: As used in stitching peritoneum, skin, etc.

2. *Curve*

a. Straight needles (may be big or small), e.g. skin needle, intestinal needle
b. Semicurved needle (may be big or small), e.g. as used in stitching peritoneum, scalp of the head, etc.

c. Half circle needle (may be big or small), e.g. Intestinal needles, VVF needles, Facia needles, Needles used in stitching uterus, cervix, etc.

3. *According to Use*

According to the area of use the needles may be:
a. Round bodied needles, e.g. intestinal needles eye needles, etc.
b. Round bodied tip cutting needles, e.g. cervix needles.
c. Cutting needles straight or curved, e.g. fascia needles, skin needles, etc.

For soft tissues, round bodied needles big or small may be used and for thick areas like skin and sole of the, leg, etc. tip cutting or full cutting needles big or small may be used. The number and size of needles required for particular operations depends upon the size of the patient, type of area and the thickness of the tissue to be stitched. The nurse has to use her own intelligence and the choice of the surgeon in selecting the type of needles for particular operations.

ANEURYSM NEEDLE

It is devised for ligating the aneurysm. The suture material is inserted to the eye of the needle and the tip of the needle is passed behind the aneurysm. The ligature thus passed is tied to exclude the aneurysm.

Features

1. It is a blunt tipped instrument which resembles a hook. The blunt tip avoids any injury to surrounding tissues.
2. The tip has got an eye and it may be curved laterally or at right angles to the shaft of the instrument.
3. The eye of the needle is preceded by a groove for the ligature.

Uses

1. It is used for ligation of an aneurysm.
2. It may be used for ligating any vessel in continuity.
3. It is used to hook out and ligate the vein during venesection.
4. It is used to ligate the cystic duct.

8. Ligatures and Sutures

Materials used for surgical ligatures and sutures can be divided into two main groups, absorbent and non-absorbent. The absorbent materials are catgut and "Living sutures" made from tendon or fascia.

Absorbent Materials

Catgut: Catgut is made from the submucous coat of sheep's intestine, very thorough cleansing is needed before the material is send for sterilization and as the sterilization process is a long and somewhat complicated one, it is usual to buy the prepared sterilized catgut in sealed glass tubes. Very stringent supervision of its preparation in all stages is observed by the manufactures and the production of catgut for surgical use is controlled by the Therapeutic Substance Act.

The sterilization of the outside of the tubes depends on the type of fluid inside the tube. Tubes containing catgut in pure alcohol may be boiled, tubes containing a mixture of alcohol and water sterilized by immersion in a cold disinfectant solution such as Bradosol 1 percent solution for twelve hours.

The rate of absorption of catgut in the tissues depends on the method of preparation of the gut and on the type of tissue in which it is embedded. Plain catgut is absorbed on the average in ten days. Chromicized catgut may take twenty, thirty, or forty days: the type most commonly used is the "twenty-day" catgut. Sizes of catgut from '000' to 4 can be obtained: '00' is the usual size for ligatures or suturing of delicate structures sizes 2 or 3 are used for stouter or structures, such as may be required for the kidney pedicle or in gynecological surgery. Fine catgut, size '00' or '0' may be used for suturing the stomach or intestine. Size 1 and 2 are used for suturing peritoneum and muscle. Fine catgut, '000' is also occasionally used for subcuticular suture and for plastic surgery.

Living sutures: These are most often used in hernioplasty and are obtained from the patient's own tissues, either the tendon of the plantaris muscle in the leg or fascia strips from fascia lata on the outer aspect of the thigh. When fascia strips are cut from the patient, it is kept in cold normal saline solution till it is used. *No antiseptics added.*

Non-absorbent Materials

Non-absorbent materials are silkworm gut, nylon thread, linen thread, silk thread, metals such as silver, aluminium and stainless steel wire and metal skin clips. Plastic or metal sachets containing sterilized sutures are prepared by surgical supply firms.

Silkworm gut is obtained from the glands of the silkworm. The material is drawn out into threads measuring about 12 inches (30 cm) in length and is made in four thickness: fine, medium, strong and extra strong. It is often dyed pink or bright purple. The strands are kept together by putting them through a piece of tubing or a metal holder. Silkworm gut is used for skin sutures and is preferably to thread as it is non-permeable. It is sterilized by boiling for five minutes.

Nylon thread: Braided or monofilament, is similar in appearance and properties to silkworm gut and is sterilized in the same way. Nylon will disintegrate in phenol.

Linen thread: May be used for ligatures in place of catgut and some surgeons use thread for intestinal and muscle sutures. It is obtained on reels in various sizes, 90, 60, 35 and 25 being the sizes most commonly used. The thread is wound on metal bobbins and boiled for thirty minutes for the first boiling and subsequently with the instruments for five minutes or autoclaved as dressings.

Silk thread: In various sizes, from the very fine silk used in arterial sutures and ophthalmic surgery. Thick silk is used for the ligation of stout structures such as a patent ductus arteriosus. Also used for a great many purposes in surgery. It can be sterilized in the same way as linen thread, but a convenient method for preparing a number of fine silk sutures, as for example, in the requirements of neurosurgery, is to thread the needles with appropriate lengths of silk in the different sizes and to darn these on to gauze pads which are sterilized by autoclaving.

"Serum proofed" silk is also used in neurosurgery and may be prepared by waxing the silk thread with Horsley's wax or may be bought ready prepared from the manufacturers. It may be prepared in the theater by winding the silk on metal winders placing in a container with melted wax, removing the silk when saturated and drying it on a sterile towel. The needles are then threaded, as described above, on to gauze pads which are placed in a drum and autoclaved. Black silk is used for the waxed and ordinary sutures in neurosurgery.

Floss silk: Purchased readymade for use in glass tubes, has a particular use in hernioplasty in place of living sutures. The tubes are sterilized by boiling.

Metal: Silver and steel wire and clips are used for various purposes. Wire filigree and wire gauze may be used for hernia repairs. The metal screws and pins used in orthopedic surgery may also be considered as a type of suture. Where metal is embedded in the tissues it is important that two different types of metal are not used as in such circumstances the tissue fluids can set up an electrolytic action with damaging results.

Ligatures of flattened silver wire are used in neurosurgery and also in lung surgery for clipping blood vessels. The short lengths of wire are cut in to a 'V' shape by special clippers. They are placed on a rest, from which they are removed by special forceps and handedover to the surgeon. These clips are known as Cushing's clips.

Metal skin clips, such as Michel's and Kifa's are used where healing of the skin is rapid, e.g. in the neck, and are also use in conjunction with tension sutures for closing an abdominal incision. All types of metal clips and wire are sterilized by boiling with the instrument required for the particular operation.

9. Syringes and Glass Wares

Record syringes and other glass and metal types are usually sterilized by boiling unless a special heat-resisting cement has been used in their construction, when they may be autoclaved. All glass syringes can be sterilized by dry heat or by autoclaving. Glass and metal syringes must first be taken apart. Otherwise the rapid expansion of the metal on heating will cause the piston to crack the glass barrel. The same precaution is necessary after use when the syringes are boiled after washing. It is important to see that pistons and barrel are checked for perfect fitness when reassembled. Syringes and needles cannot be efficiently sterilized by chemical means.

Glass ampoules containing drugs should be autoclaved, unless specific directions to the contrary are given by the doctor who will administer drug. If these ampoules are placed in a disinfectant solution there is considerable danger of the solution penetrating through an undetected crack in the glass.

Other glass articles are sterilized in the methods used for syringes.

Glass wares should not be boiled with heavy instruments or linen. They should be wrapped in old linen or cotton to protect it from damage against the sides of the sterilizers.

10. Enamel and Other Metal Ware

Bowls, trays, gallipots and receivers are sterilized by autoclaving or boiling. They should be arranged by sizes in such a manner that one utensil does not stick inside another forming a pocket of air which will prevent thorough penetration of the heat during the sterilizing process.

After use, bowls, gallipots and other articles are washed and any stains are removed by the use of cleaning powder.

11. Nail Brushes

New brushes are boiled for thirty minutes and are reboiled for five minutes or autoclaved between cases.

They are usually dished dry into sterile bowls or boxes.

5 Common Technical Terms

Definitions of some of the commoner suffixes may help the nurse to understand strange, and often alarmingly long words although it must be stated that these word endings are not always used correctly and that in some instances incorrect terminology is sanctioned by common usage.

-ectomy: A suffix denoting removal or excision of a structure, e.g. hysterectomy, removal of the uterus.

-orrhaphy: A plastic or repair operation, e.g. perineorrhaphy repair of the perineum. The ending 'plasty' is also used to describe a plastic operation where the aim is to rebuild and restore tissues destroyed by injury or disease.

-oscopy: Inspection of the interior of an organ or passage by means of special instruments, usually carrying a light, e.g. cystoscopy, examination of the bladder by means of cystoscope.

-ostomy: Constructing an artificial opening into an organ, e.g. gastrostomy marking an opening from the stomach on to the surface of the abdomen.

-otomy: incising or dividing a structure, e.g. laparotomy—incising and opening the abdomen; tenotomy—dividing a tendon.

It is the use of the last two terms that inaccuracies are most commonly found, for example, the operation of making an opening into the trachea in order to insert a tube is correctly called 'tracheostomy' but is quite frequently referred to as 'tracheotomy'.

Antrostomy: Making an opening in to the maxillary antrum to provide drainage. The most extensive type of antrostomy is known as Caldwell-Luc's operation.

Appendicectomy: Removal of the appendix.

Appendicostomy: Establishing an opening between the lumen of the appendix and the abdominal wall for the purpose of irrigating the colon.

Arthrodesis: An operation to stiffen a joint permanently and prevent movement.

Arthroplasty: An operation designed to increase the amount of movement at a joint.

Arthrotomy: Making an opening into a joint for drainage or exploration.

Bronchoscopy: Inspection of the interior of the bronchial tree by means of a bronchoscope. Draining an abscess, removal of a foreign body or of a section of a growth may all be carried out as part of a bronchoscopy.

Cesarean section: Removal of the fetus, at or near term from the uterus by an abdominal incision.

Cholecystectomy: Removal of the gallbladder.

Cholecystenterostomy: Establishing an opening between the gallbladder and the small intestine. Cholecystogastrostomy is a similar operation connecting the gallbladder and the stomach. These operations are performed to provide drainage of the bile into the alimentary tract when the common bile duct is permanently obstructed, as for example, by the pressure of a growth in the head of the pancreas.

Cholecystotomy: Opening the gallbladder.

Choledochotomy: Opening the common bile duct.

Chordotomy: Division of nerve tracts within the spinal cord.

Colostomy: Making an opening into the colon to act as a temporary or permanent anus for the discharge of feces. The usual sites are the descending and transverse colon.

Cecostomy is the term used when the opening is made into the cecum.

Colporrhaphy: A repair operation on the vaginal wall in the treatment of pelvic prolapse. Stretching of the anterior vaginal wall and prolapse of the uterus may allow the bladder and urethra to bulge into the vaginal canal, producing the condition known as a cystocele; for this, the operation of anterior colporrhaphy is performed. A similar condition of the posterior vaginal wall producing a rectocele is dealt with by the operation of posterior colporrhaphy. Both these operations may be combined with perineorrhaphy.

Craniotomy: Opening the cavity of the skull, as for example, for the removal of a tumor, draining an abscess, or in the treatment of cranial injuries.

Cystectomy: Excision of the urinary bladder.

Cystoscopy: Inspection of the interior of the bladder by means of cystoscope passed through urethra. Catheterization of the ureters, cauterizing papillomata, (fulguration) and resection of the prostate glands may be carried out via an operating cystoscope.

Curettage: Removing tissues by scraping with a curette or spoon. The term is most commonly used for removal of overgrown lymphatic tissues (adenoids) in the nasopharynx and for curettage of the interior of the uterus.

Diathermy: A high-frequency electric current producing great heat. In surgery diathermy is used for cautery and as the 'diathermy knife' which seals the vessels as it cuts.

Ectopic gestation: Implantation and development of a fertilized ovum outside the cavity of the uterus, usually in a fallopian tube. A ruptured ectopic gestation is a condition that usually required urgent operation.

Embolectomy: Removal of an embolus from an artery or vein. Pulmonary embolectomy is also known as Trendelenburg's operation.

Epididymectomy: Excision of the epididymis, a series of tubules lying behind the testes and continuous with the vasdeference.

Episiotomy: Incision of the perineum in the second stage of labor to prevent extensive laceration.

Gastrectomy: Excision of the stomach. Total removal is a rare operation. The usual operation is a partial gastrectomy.

Gastroenterostomy: Making an anastomosis between the stomach and the small intestine, usually the jejunum. Following this operation the stomach contents bypass the pyloric end of the stomach and duodenum; therefore it is sometimes referred to as 'short-circuiting'.

Gastroscopy: Inspection of the mucous lining of the stomach using a flexible gastroscope.

Gastrostomy: Making an artificial opening into the stomach for the purpose of feeding a patient having an esophageal stricture.

Gastrotomy: Opening the stomach for exploration or removal of a foreign body.

Hydrocele: A collection of fluid in the tunica vaginalis of the scrotum.

Hymenectomy: Excising and trimming an imperforate or rigid hymen.

Hysterectomy: Removal of the uterus. A subtotal hysterectomy implies removal of the body of the uterus leaving the cervix.

Total hysterectomy: Removal of the entire uterus.

Pan-hysterectomy: Removal of the uterus, Fallopian tubes and ovaries.

Radical or Wertheim's hysterectomy: Removal of the uterus, appendages, upper part of the vagina and adjacent connective tissue.

Herniotomy: Operation for the repair of hernia.

Ileostomy: Making an opening into the ileum.

Iridectomy: Removal of section of the iris of the eye as a preliminary to cataract extraction or for the relief of tension in glaucoma.

Jejunostomy: Making an opening into the jejunum.

Laminectomy: Cutting through and removing the laminae of the vertebral column, as for example, in operations for a prolapsed intervertebral disc, as an approach to the spinal cord, e.g. for removal of a tumor.

Laparotomy: Opening the abdominal cavity. A varying number of conditions which come under the heading of the 'acute abdomen' may be the reason for an emergency laparotomy, e.g. acute appendicitis, acute cholecystitis, intestinal obstruction, as for example, strangulated hernia intussusception, malignant growth or volvulus.

Laryngectomy: Removal of the larynx.

Laryngoscopy: Inspection of the interior of the larynx by a mirror and reflected light is indirect laryngoscopy, or by means of laryngoscope is direct laryngoscopy.

Laryngofissure: Splitting the thyroid cartilage of the larynx to expose the vocal cords.

Laryngostomy: Opening the larynx and introducing laryngostomy tube, an operation sometimes performed in cases of extreme urgency when the glottis is blocked. NB the terms 'laryngotomy' and 'tracheotomy' are in common use for the operations of introducing a tube into the larynx or trachea although the correct terms are 'laryngostomy' and 'tracheostomy'.

Leucotomy: Division of some of the white nerve fibers in the frontal area of the brain. The operation is most commonly performed for the relief of mental conditions associated with extreme emotional tension or anxiety.

Litholapaxy or Lithotrity: Crushing a vesicle calculus by means of an instrument known as a lithotrite introduced per urethra.

Lobectomy: Removal of a lobe of the lung.

Mastectomy: Removal of the breast, radical mastectomy denotes removal of the breast, the underlying pectoral muscles and adjacent lymph glands in the treatment of the breast.

Meniscectomy: Removal of a cartilage in the knee joint, an operation performed for the condition known as internal derangements of the knee joint (IDK).

Myomectomy: Removal of a fibromyoma or "fibroid" from the uterus.

Myringotomy: Incision of the tympanic membrane of the ear to drain the middle ear. This operation is also known as paracentesis tympani.

Nephrectomy: Removal of a kidney.

Nephropexy: Suturing kidney to the posterior abdominal wall, to fix it in normal position.

Nephrostomy: Establishing an opening into the pelvis of the kidney for the purpose of drainage.

Nephrotomy: Incising the kidney, usually for the removal of a renal calculus. This operation is also known as "nephrolithotomy".

Esophagoscopy: Examination of the interior of the esophagus as a diagnostic procedure or for the removal of a foreign body.

Oophorectomy: Removal of one or both ovaries. The older term "ovariectomy" is also used.

Overiostomy: Making an opening in a ovarian cyst for drainage purpose.

Overiotomy: Making an incision into or removal of an ovary or removal of a tumor of the ovary.

Orchidectomy: Removal of the testis.

Osteotomy: Division of a bone to correct a deformity or as part of an arthroplastic operation. The instrument used is an osteotome differs from chisel. In that it is bevelled on both side.

Perineorrhaphy: Repair of the perineum. The term is used for the repair carried out when prolapse of the uterus has occurred as a result of a weakened pelvic floor and is not usually used for the simple suturing of a lacerated perineum performed immediately after labor.

Pharyngotomy: Opening the pharynx to gain access to a malignant growth of the upper part of the esophagus. As the approach is from the side, the operation is known as "lateral pharyngotomy".

Phrenic avulsion: Tearing the fibers of the phrenic nerve from their attachment to the diaphragm, producing paralysis of one dome of the diaphragm and collapse of the lower part of the lung on that side. The approach to the nerve is made through a small incision in the neck division of the nerve is carried out in addition to avulsion.

Pneumonectomy: Removal of one lung in the radical treatment of bronchiectasis, tuberculosis, or malignant disease of the lung.

Pneumothorax: Air in pleural space. The operation, referred to as an "extrapleural" pneumothorax, involves injecting air between the pleura and the chest wall after stripping off the parietal pleura.

Prostatectomy: Removal of the prostate gland, which lies at the base of the bladder in the male, usually through a transvesical, suprapubic or retropubic incision. Transurethral resection of the prostate gland is carried out by diathermy.

Pyelolithotomy: Removal of a stone from the pelvis of the kidney.

Pyelogram (Retrograde): X-ray examination of the renal pelvis, after the injection of a radiopaque medium via ureteric catheters.

Rammstedt's operation: Incising the muscular coat of the stomach at the pyloric end for the relief of pyloric stenosis in infants.

Splenectomy: Removal of the spleen. Traumatic rupture of the spleen is a common reason for its removal, but the operation may also be performed in certain disease of the blood.

Tarsorrhaphy: Suturing the eyelids together to protect the eye.

Thoracoplasty: Opening the chest cavity, e.g. to drain an empyema or repair of abnormalities or defects in the thorax.

Thoracectomy: Removal of several ribs on one side of the chest to produce collapse of the underlying lung in the treatment of tuberculosis. It is also called thoracotomy that is incision of the chest wall.

Thoracoscopy: Examination of the pleural space by means of a thoracoscope inserted through the chest wall.

Trachelorrhaphy: The operation for the repair of a lacerated cervix.

Tracheostomy: Opening the trachea and introducing a tracheostomy tube. In the usual operation the trachea is opened at the level of the thyroid gland. The operation referred to as a "high" tracheostomy may be performed in emergencies, the opening being made through the upper rings of the trachea which are close to the skin surface.

Trephining: Removal of a disc of tissue, usually applied to the removal of a disc of bone from the skull, but is also used for the operation of removing a small disc of the sclerotic coat of the eye in case of chronic glaucoma.

Ureterolithotomy: The operation of opening the ureter to remove a calculus.

Urethrotomy: Incising the urethra for the relief of stricture. Internal urethrotomy is the term used for the operation of slitting the stricture with a guarded knife passed into the urethra. External urethrotomy implies opening the urethra from the outside, the incision being made through the perineum.

Ventriculography: Radiography of the cerebral ventricles after removal of cerebrospinal fluid and its replacement by air introduced via a hollow needle. Trephine holes are made in the skull through which the needles are passed.

Ventrosuspension: The term is usually used for the operation of shortening the round ligaments of the uterus, which run forward to the inguinal canal, suspending the uterus in the anteverted position. Gilliam's is the most common type of this operation.

Vesical: Relating to the urinary bladder.

Vulvectomy: Excision of the vulva.

6. Role of the Nurses in Major Operations

ROLE OF A NURSE IN THE CONDUCT OF A MAJOR ABDOMINAL OPERATION

Scrubbed Nurse

- Washing the hands thoroughly.
- Putting the sterile cap and mask.
- Scrubbing the hands up to elbow for 5 mts to 10 mts (as detailed under scrubbing).
- Dipping the hands in the lotion in the vertical lotion jar.
- Wiping the hands with sterile towel.
- Putting the sterile gown as detailed under gowning.
- Fixing the sleeves at the wrists.
- Rubbing in and outside of the palms with rectified spirit.
- Putting the sterile gloves as detailed under gloving and wash the gloved hands in sterile water or lotion to remove the powder.

(Meanwhile one running nurse or technician see that the patient is kept safe on the operation table) One doctor will be anesthetising and starting the IV drip of suitable solution in time and changing the position of the patient on the table according to the type of operation. Any change of position of the table is made with the permission of the anesthetist.

During this period the other running nurse or technician supply the sterile caps, masks, gowns, spirit and gloves, first to the assistant doctor.

(The works of the instrument nurse and running person are going on simultaneously).

Instrument nurse continues her procedure. Reaching in between the patient on the table and the trolley which is carbolised already.

Spreads the sterile sheet and tray cover, (tray over the oepration table is fitted on the Mayo stand).

Adjust the Mayo stand over the patient at the foot end and keep the instrument for the immediate use only in it Running person handles all the sterile set of instruments, drapings, mops, suture materials and other required items either from the drum or by transfer forceps. Usually one complete set is prepared in one drum or packet.

Instrument nurse washes the gloved hands in sterile water again before touching the sterile instruments. Arrange the instruments according to the order of use in the tray adjusted over the patient. Counts the instruments which are more in number, e.g. artery forceps. *Counts the Mops and instruct the running person to Mark in on the Board. Counts the needles and other multiple items.* Break the catguts and fix them on needles and mount them in needle holders according to the situation required. Keep ready the ligatures. Mount the cotton swabs on sponge holders ready to dip in antiseptic lotion for cleaning the area for operation.

Meanwhile the surgeon and assistant approaches the patient and get the permission of the anesthetist to start the operation. Anesthetist agrees to start the operation means that the patient is under anesthesia. Surgeon and assistant wash the gloved hands in sterile water which is kept near the table, separate for both. One of the runner expose the field of operation by removing the clothes and binder of the patient on that area and adjust the shadowless lamp. Instrument nurse handles the cotton sponges soaked in antiseptic, held on the sponge holders. Usually two or three times this cleaning is repeated followed by a swabbing with rectified spirit swab. These sponge holders are discarded. Spreads the drapings with the help of the surgeon according to the area to be operated. Handle the towel clips to the surgeon to fix the drapings. Handle the knife and skin mops. Wet mops are more absorbable. Pass on the artery forceps and mops to the assistant to catch the bleeding points while the surgeon opens the skin (some time electric cautery may be used). Or supply the ligatures either plain catgut or cotton thread to tie the bleeding points, while handling the suture cutting scissors to the assistant. When all the bleeding points are cleared all the instruments and mops used are received in a sterile kidney tray and removed from the field of operation and kept at the side of the instrument trolley. Instrument nurse, surgeon and assistants wash their hands in fresh sterile water or even changes their gloves. Separate sterile bowls are kept for each one which are replenished by the runners as required. Instrument nurse supply the skin towels and skin clips. Adjust the instrument trolley and Mayo stand more conveniently. Supply another knife for cutting the fascia and a pair of scissors to extend the cut according to the skin incision. With the distal end of the knife-handle the muscles are separated but not cut. Two Alley's forceps are given to lift the peritoneum so that the intestinal contents are not injured while opening the abdomen. Knife is given to make a small opening in between the two Alley's forceps, which is enlarged by scissors. Retractors are given to the surgeon. Mops are supplied as required and a wet abdominal pack, which is larger than the mops to cover the contents other than the organ to be handled, is given. The instrument nurse should be very careful to see that the tape hanging on the mops and the pack are extended to the outside of the opening so that they are not missed inside. Sometimes artery forceps are clamped in these tapes. The instruments and ligatures are handled according to the situation as far as possible anticipating the needs during the actual session of operation. Meanwhile she should concentrate her attention that all the instruments, mops and needles are kept only outside the cavity when not in actual use but provide easiness of handling these to the surgeon and assistant. When mops are soiled, replace them. Time for the work of the surgeon varies according to the type of operation and skill of the surgeon. The anesthetist is keenly watching the general condition of the patient. Even though the observation of the surgeons and the instrument nurse will do only good to the patient. Any change of color in the oozing blood in the site of operation is an indication of lack of oxygen to the patient and deterioration from the normal. If such change is noted during operation, it should be brought to the notice of the anesthetist immediately.

When the actual session of operation is finished the surgeon takes off the instruments from the site. The instrument nurse removes all the instruments, mops and needles to the trolley making sure that all the articles are correct to the counting as per the number as it was before starting the operation. Clear the field by removing all the bits of catguts and ligatures and spread a fresh towel over the previous drapings. Supply a fresh mop to the surgeon to clean the cavity and its organs which may prevent the future formation of adhesions, to a certain extent. Then receive the pack from inside which is kept by the surgeon. The surgeon keeps the abdominal contents in their normal position.

Before supplying the materials for closing the abdomen make *sure once again that all the instruments, needles, pack and mops are removed out and correct to the counting marked on the board before operation* and convince the surgeon. The instrument nurse should be extremely alert and concentrate in her work during operation to prevent any mishappening in this matter. When everything is seen alright she may proceed to supply the articles for closing the abdomen.

Supply Alley's forceps as required number to hold the peritoneum. Give catgut No. 1 on a round bodied half circle needle held on needle holder, a toothed dissecting forceps to the surgeon and suture cutting scissors to the assistant.

Mops given as required. In case of stitching the peritoneum No. 1 or No. 'O' catgut with a round bodied needle held on needle holder is given. Some surgeons prefer to put some interrupted sutures on reflected muscles and others replace them in normal position.

Then Kocher's forceps or Alley's tissue forceps are given to hold the fascia in apposition. When they are approximated, the assistant will hold them in place. The surgeon receives the cutting half circle needles with chro: catgut No.1 or No.2 in sufficient length, on the needle holder and start stitching. A toothed dissecting forceps is in his left hand.

When the stitching is progressing the Kocher's forceps are removed and finally the assistant cuts off the tips of the sutures at both ends. Then the surgeon removes the skin towels and skin clips and the incisional area is cleaned with a fresh swab.

By this time the instrument nurse prepares the Alley's forceps to hold the skin in apposition and the tip cutting straight skin needle with cotton thread or any skin suture materials according to the preference of the surgeon. These materials are given to the surgeon and the suture cutting scissors to the assistant. During the time of skin suturing, the instrument nurse clear off the field and tray by removing all the instruments, balance of suture materials, needles, mops, etc. and hand over to the runner who takes them to the utility room for cleaning, etc.

After stitching the skin, the drapings and towel clips are removed with the help of the surgeon or assistant while the nurse is covering the wound with a fresh mop with one hand.

When every thing is removed from the actual field, the area around the wound is cleaned by using plenty of rectified spirit soaked in cotton swabs held on a forceps. Apply the thick pad of abdominal dressing and fix them in position either by binder or adhesive plaster.

The anesthetist remove the endotracheal tube, etc. from the patient except the air way which is kept in the mouth. Keep the hands of the patient at the sides of the body. The instrument nurse replaces clean dresses to the patient. Anesthetist and the surgeon checks the general condition of the patient.

If the general condition is normal they give permission to the nurse to shift the patient from the table to the trolley. She with the help of the assistants changes the patient to the trolley by holding the bottle of IV drip without slipping from the vein. The surgeon, assistant and the instrument nurse remove their gloves, gowns, mops and masks and keep them in their proper places. Surgeon writes the immediate postoperative instructions in the chart and entrust it to the instrument nurse. The operation notes are entered in the register and the surgeon anesthetist, assistant and the instrument nurse put their signatures in the register.

The face of the patient is wiped to remove the stain of adhesive plaster and the smell of anesthetic drugs, to a certain extent. The patient on the trolley is shifted to the ward or recovery room accompanied by one of the running nurses and entrusted to the sister in charge of the ward or recovery room, along with the case sheet. The sister in charge receives the patient on the bed, noting the general condition of the patient and the time of arrival. She accepts the case sheet to note the immediate postoperative instructions and by this, the responsibility of the theater nurse is over about that particular patient. The trolley attender returns the trolley to the theater along with the linen and blanket which are used to cover the patient on transportation.

The instrument nurse and the other running nurse see the cleaning and replenishing of operation table, trolleys, trays, drums, etc. to start the next operation.

SPECIAL POINTS

During operations, the instrument nurse handles the instrument to the surgeon as far as possible anticipating the need.

The mops and the suture cutting scissors are handed over to the assistant at his disposal. During operation complete silence is maintained in the operation room. Catguts and other suture materials are taken to sufficient length at the time of use without much wastage.

Needles are selected according to the tissue of the area for use.

The running nurses or technicians are always at the call of the instrument nurse and anesthetist for help. They should be alert in changing the hand lotions as required, counting the mops, supplying any extra sterile instruments, etc.

These should be the system of routine work in the operation room before and after the operation. Every member should work with the team spirit for the successful functioning of the operation room simultaneously. The given procedure of the operation is for major abdominal operation of an adult patient. The usual steps before and after are same for every operation. But the selection of instruments, drapings, needles and ligatures varies in size, type and in number according to the type of operation and the size of the patient. The principles and techniques are same for every operation with slight differences.

Surgery may be done for a variety of reasons; to remove foreign body, to remove diseased parts, to correct deformities, to repair poorly functioning parts, to diagnose the disease or for exploratory purpose. Whatever, be the reason, all precautions are taken to handle the tissues gently and carefully. The incision will easily heal when it is a clean smooth cut. For adequate exposure and minimum trauma from retractors, the incision should be adequate. The knife must be sharp enough to prevent an irregular incision.

The process of controlling hemorrhage is called hemostasis which is an important part of the operation because it prevents blood loss and shock, lessen the occurrence of postoperative hematoma and enable the surgeon to dissect more accurately in a bloodless area. In order to make the operation field dry and visible, sponges for moping or other control means are used. When an assistant or scrubbing nurse use sponge in a wound it must be used to blot by gentle pressure, as rubbing or using force injures delicate tissues.

Salient Responsibilities of the Scrubbed Nurse

Before going for scrubbing, she should see that the circulating nurse is preparing everything for the operation. If time allows she can help the circulating person for preparation. When it is time she scrubs hands and puts the sterile cap, mask, gown and gloves and washes her gloved hands in sterile water.

- Arrange the instruments according to the order of use on the sterile trolley so that they are readily accessible.
- Place knife blades on handles.
- Count the sponges with circulating nurse.
- Arrange suture materials and prepare ligatures and sutures as required.
- Check the articles immediately before use especially materials which are liable to get in disorder or inside the abdomen at any time, e.g. suction tips, suture needles, forceps, etc.
- Cover the sterile articles on the sterile table with a sterile towel until the patient is anesthetised and the surgeon is ready to drape the operating field.

- Supply the instruments and other articles to the surgeon and assistant by observing the operative procedure and anticipating their needs.
- Observe the color of the blood oozing from the patient to note any lack of oxygen and if any, it should be reported to the surgeon and anesthetist because any amount of observation will do only good to the patient even though it is the responsibility of the anesthetist.

Individual surgeons have individual preferences in their operative procedures. The scrubbed nurse should learn how to work best with him as a smooth working team member. She can learn to supply the articles by anticipating intelligently the needs only by watching the field of operation and understanding the progress of operation. She is responsible for keeping the field neat by arranging the instruments, removing the bits of sutures and ligatures and replacing the unnecessary instruments. The nurses working in the operation theatre should develop the skill by their practice, observation and by the guidance from expert seniors and earnest workmanship.

Responsibilities of the Circulating Nurse during a Major Operation

The circulating nurse has many responsibilities during an operation. She should anticipate and meet the needs of the scrubbed nurse, surgeon and anesthetist. Along with that, she is responsible for the safety and comfort of the patient as any other person. Under no condition is she permitted to leave the room unless she is replaced. Some of her activities include the following:
- Arrange to bring the patient from the premedication room and place on the operation table safely from the trolley when it is time.
- See that the techniques are maintained properly without break.
- Assume responsibility with other members of the team for the comfort and safety of the patient.
- Keep the scrubbed nurse supplied with dressing, suture materials, etc.

- Attach the suction apparatus and see that it is in working condition and assist the anesthetist when required.
- Adjust the buckets to receive the discarded sponges.
- Retrive instruments, etc. which accidentally fall from the table.
- Replace saline or water in basins as necessary, near the surgeons instrument nurse and assistant doctor.
- Regulate temperature of the room as necessary.
- Count the sponges with scrubbed nurse and see that no sponge is taken away from the room during an abdominal operation.
- Adjust the shadowless lamp or spot light in position.
- Adjust the position of the table during operation with the permission of the anesthetist and as required.
- Take care of specimens.
- Prepare adhesive plaster, scissors, binder or bandage for securing the dressing following the wound closure, if it is the practice.
- See that the patient is safely transferred to the recovery room after operation.
- Direct the cleaning and preparation of the room for the next operation.
- From these responsibilities it is evident that a circulating nurse should be prepared for that position.
- She should possess the ability to organise activities and direct personnel with due understanding of interpersonal relationship.
- She should have the ability to anticipate the needs of that situation.
- She should have the ability to differentiate between situations which demand immediate attention and those of lesser importance.
- Ability to maintain a quiet, neat and well equipped unit.
- She should understand thoroughly the principles of asepsis.
- She should have the ability to teach the members of the team and set example to them.
- She should be alert and respond to any happening in the operation room.

Procedure Following a Contaminated Operation

A contaminated or dirty case is an operation in which pus or gangrene is found. If it is a planned operation, it should be done only as the last case of the day; that is after all the clean cases are over. The care of articles used for dirty case differs very little from the so called clean cases. The basic principle is that all contaminated articles, gowns, gloves, instruments, sponges and drapes must be handled as little as possible as they are prepared and transported to the sterilizer or place of disposition. They should be disposed immediately. It is better that one person remains to receive all soiled linen and other articles in a special bag marked 'contaminated'. All the gloves used for that particular operation should be collected and washed in one basin to prevent mingling of other basins and other gloves. All the rubber articles used should be sterilized together in a washer sterilizer. Instruments should not be mingled with other instruments and boiled separately. Needles should be collected in a metal needle box and autoclaved. Glass suture tubes should be washed in cold water and immersed in any germicide. Unused sponges, dressings and linen are received in a dry linen bag and autoclaved. Soiled sponges and other discarded items are collected in paper bag before being transported to the incinerator. Solutions and suction bottle contents are emptied in a bucket and disposed into the proper place. Instrument table and operating table, buckets and other utensils are scrubbed thoroughly with a germicide. As far as possible used linen or any other dirty materials should not touch the floor.

If the septic areas and articles are cleansed thoroughly and sterilized or disposed off, the room may be prepared for the next case. It is not necessary to quarantine the room. The floor and the walls are moped with germicide lotion with particular attention to the area where there is any spot of pus or blood. When the patient with tuberculosis comes to the operating room he should wear a mask. Intubation tubes and anesthesia face masks following their use on a patient with tuberculosis should be scrubbed inside and out with a solution of chlorinated lime (4 tsp to a gallon of water) before sending for sterilization.

Instruments, sponges and all other articles used for a gastrointestinal surgery will be dirty and even contaminated. They should be cleaned separately and carefully sterilized as it has come in contact with contents of the intestine. Gowns and gloves need special attention as for a dirty case.

CARE OF SPECIMENS

A specimen is any tissue removed from the patient during operation. Most specimens are sent for the pathological examination whereas culture, spinal fluids, urine and smears are sent to the bacteriology laboratory. When any nurse is posted to the operation room she should have an orientation of the usual procedure about the specimen, followed in the particular hospital. She must realize that the future of many patients is dependant upon the result of the laboratory studies of a small specimen of tissues. So nurse's responsibility for safeguarding and caring for the specimen is a real and great one. Her responsibility is two fold that: (1) The specimen must be labeled properly and (2) It must be sent to the proper laboratory and in time. Each specimen should be handled carefully so as not to destroy any natural land marks or characteristic which aid in the diagnosis. Specimen should be kept in a container with sufficient amount of water or saline. Allowing the specimen to dry causes autolyses and the specimen becomes useless for study. There are several exceptions to this general rule. So the nurse should be familiar with policies of the individual hospitals and laboratories. For example, specimens for frozen sections are taken to the laboratory immediately they are obtained. Specimens obtained by D and C is washed to remove the excess of blood, with citrate solution before they are kept in formalin. Smears are placed in equal parts of 95% alcohol and ether. In some places, tissue specimens are put directly in formalin as soon as they are obtained. The nurses in the operating room must adhere to the existing rules about the specimen. Keep it with proper label, sent them to the proper place and keep record of it for the future references. She should be always conscious that no patient should suffer the ill-effects resulting from the negligence of the theater people about keeping and sending the specimen.

PREMEDICATION ROOM

Premedication of an operation means the drug given to the patient before he is taken to the operation table. Considering the physical and mental relaxation of the patient before operation, he is allowed to lie in a room after the administration of drug, in the theater block which is called premedication room. It is realized as one of the essential part of the modern operation room. Patient is brought from the ward in a trolley with all the relevant records in time and allowed to be in the premedication room. Changing the cloth of the patient with theater garment as soon as he is brought from the ward is an efficient method of preventing contamination, if possible. Usually the anesthetist will be examining the patient in the ward in the previous evening and instructions are written in the chart according to the anesthesia. In some cases premedication is given in the ward before the patient is taken to the premedication room. The time of giving injection depends upon the instruction given by the anesthetist. Till the time that the patient is shifted to the table, he should be kept under close observation. Relatives are not allowed in that room but it is required that one nurse should be made responsible for the care of the patients in that room.

Patients are not allowed to walk after premedication. So the personal needs are to be attended in the bed itself, if required. Most of them will be sleepy after the injection, as sedatives are included to relieve the anxiety. Patients who are waiting for longer period without sleep even after injection may feel to pass urine or motion or vomit even though it is not needed physically. In such cases receptacles for the same should be easily accessible in the adjacent room, BP apparatus is a 'must' in that room.

Usually the members of the anesthetic team are responsible for the care and observation of the patients in the premedication room. Still the theatre sister should see that one nurse is responsible for the care of patients in that room.

RECOVERY ROOM

Recovery stage means the immediate postoperative period or the time taken by the patient to come out from the effect of anesthesia by which the vital functions of the patients returns to normal. The importance of close observations of the anesthetist, surgeon and the required efficient nursing care during this period are the basis for the establishment of a recovery room attached to the operation room. So, that room should be equipped with all the articles required to meet any immediate postoperative or postanesthetic emergencies. One efficient nurse should be in charge of that room.

The important articles required in that room include: O_2 cylinder in good working condition, suction apparatus with connections in order, BP apparatus, saline stands and trolley containing sufficient bottles of IV fluids, arm board, bandage, adhesive plaster, scissors, sterile syringes for injections, emergency drugs, transfer forceps, spirits ammonia in bottle, spirit for cleaning skin before injection, cotton swabs, forceps, tongue clips, tongue forceps, mouth gag, airways, kidney tray, tourniquet, blankets, sheets, pulse and BP chart, white paper and pen (red and blue), scale and pencil, etc. Temperature tray should be kept in the trolley.

The vital signs are observed and charted till he is shifted to the ward. Surgeon and anesthetist visit the patient as required and with their permission he is changed from the theater trolley to the ward trolley; patient is accompanied by a nurse who came from the ward, with the chart and operation notes, noting the time and conditions of the patient, on it. When the patient is entrusted to the ward nurse, the responsibility of theater nurse is over about that particular patient.

7. Prevention of Contamination in Operation Room

The success of any operation depends upon many factors such as proper preoperative care, health status and stage of disease of the patient, standard of aseptic technique followed in the operation room, ability of the surgeon and the efficient postoperative care given to the patient. Many people are involved in the project and each one's role is equally important in the case of individual patient. Maintaining high standard of aseptic technique is the responsibility of the theater nurse. It does not confine to a single person's responsibility or a single procedure in the theater. But the quality of the work going on for a particular task in the unit considerably depends upon the efficiency and technical competency of the leader. So, Sister in charge of the theater is the keynote to organize and maintain a proper aseptic condition of an operation room. Her role in this matter is very elaborate and it is impossible to explain it in detail. Still the following points will serve as a guide for the nurses working in the operation room.

The theater Sister should be a specially trained person in the subject and she should be an efficient and experienced one. She should possess some extra qualities along with her qualifications. She should be strict enough to establish and maintain all the conditions to prevent any source of contamination and to practice the principles of disinfections and sterilization. She should teach and set example to other workers and encourage them to follow the principles of cleanliness, disinfection and sterilization wherever and whenever required in the theater. Once in a way, she should arrange study classes with all the workers in the theater to remind them about these points.

As mentioned in the previous chapter, people working in the operation room should change their dress with theater garments (gown, cap, mask and shoes) before they start their work in the theater, every morning. When we think about the problem of infection and sepsis in the surgical cases, we have to realize that the use of sarees and bell bottom pants which sweep the floor carry more organisms than any other unsterile materials brought into the theater. All the attentions and precautionary preparations become futile by careless dress of the theater staff and medical attendants entering the sterile area. It is also noted by research that theater infection is partially due to the uncared, inattended hair of the surgeons, and nurses and housemen. It may be a remark to the hippy models, step cutting and water free styles.

Considering these facts too, it should be noted that the theater dress should be worn properly while working there. It should not be for the attraction or recognition or identification or decoration. It should serve the purpose for which it is intended. The gown should be loose enough and cover the body properly in front and back. Sleeves should be at least up to the elbow for ordinary and full sleeved after scrubbing, to fit inside the cuff of the sterile gloves. Cap for males and head towel for females should be large enough to cover the hair properly and no curles should hang in the front or back. Mask should be sufficiently large enough to cover the nose and mouth. Once a mask or cap is taken away from the face or head it should be replaced by another one to enter inside. It is a very common malpractice we see with many people that a used mask is hanging on the tape of the gown in the waist or pocket and after some time the same one is in their face which should be strictly avoided. Remember that it is contaminated when once used. Avoid or at least minimise talking inside the theater. If possible communications outside the units should be limited by telephone talk. The workers should be of clean nature and free from any diseases especially respiratory and skin conditions. The workers should not be allowed to go and wander outside the unit during their working hours and none from outside should be allowed inside without theater garments.

Our body and dress contain numerous micro-organisms which are harmless to ourselves and others in one condition. But they can produce harm in some other condition. These organisms will be distributed to air from our body without our knowledge. Spores of organisms are commonly present in the soil which will be present in our shoes when walking outside. They are also harmless to intact skin. But they will take its vegetative forms, multiply and produce serious infections when the conditions are favorable for their growth. They are easily distributed in the floor from the shoes if one walks inside without changing the shoes used outside. Because of all these reasons that theater block is separated away from the thoroughfare of the hospital. Visitors are not allowed and the workers are insisted to use only theater garments and shoes while working. This fact should be emphasised to the workers at times. Even though, there is less numbers of operation for the day, it should not be a practice to change nurses and other workers from the theater to the wards and from the wards to the theater for working arrangements. So also, visitors should not be allowed for assembling or walking in the corridor or entrance of the unit.

The construction of a modern theater is suitable for the maintenance of aseptic conditions. The different adjacent rooms should be used only for the purpose for which it is intended. By which it means, for example, a packing room should not be used as changing room for the workers or a utility room should not be used for dining room and so on. Food and drinks are not allowed to bring from outside especially from shops. Food packets brought by the workers should be eaten only in the room provided for the same and not in any other room. Minimize the chance of workers going outside the unit for food. In unavoidable circumstances they must go in their own dress but when return for work a fresh theater dress must be used. Once a dress is used and removed from the body, it should be considered as contaminated and it must be laundered properly before the next use or proper gown technique must be used. The Senior Sister must keep close observation in these matters.

Wet cleaning and carbolizing the operation table, trolleys. Mayo stand, etc. in the main room should be carefully done in the morning and this system should be followed everyday. Using mask is a 'must' while working inside. In the evening, the tyre pieces on the operation table should be taken away, washed with soap and water and dried. Table should be cleaned whenever necessary and oiled according to the instructions of makers. Spare parts should not be kept on the floor. A weekly scheduled thorough cleaning of the room and articles should be insisted. The care of operation room after a contaminated operation is performed as mentioned in the previous chapter. Everyone should be instructed to minimize the handling of dirty articles and to use forceps in such conditions. Articles to be used for operation should not be allowed to put or touch on the floor. If at all, it happens it must be sterilized again before use. If it is substances like cotton or thread it should be discarded as we are not sure about the purity of the floor.

Theater linen are not washed with the ward linen in the laundry. If washing is done in the common laundry, it should be scheduled to use the laundry for washing theater linen alone for a day after thorough cleaning and disinfection of the laundry machine and room. If possible the washing is arranged in the theater block itself. This practice will prevent contamination and missing of linen and increase the durability of the material. Mops and drapes to be used for operation should not be used as covering for the packets or bundles or for cleaning purpose and vice versa. While packing linen for sterilization, it should be inspected for stains and its cleanliness. Torn or dirty material should not be used for packing. Folding should be done in such a way for the better handling without making it unsterile. Hanging or loose thread must be removed before packing. Allow free entrance of steam in between folds as well as each cloth during autoclaving, by proper packing. Linen should not be put on the floor after use and dirty linen should not be mixed with clean linen and not taken to the packing room. Clothes soaked with blood or discharge should be washed separately before it is taken for washing with other linen. Drapings used for contaminated operation should be treated by intermittent sterilization after careful laundering. Misuse or improper use of any linen should be prevented. While autoclaving, ward linen packets or any other articles from ward should not be kept in the autoclave with the theater linen. Shoe cover used by unavoidable visitors in rare instances should be washed and boiled separately and do not mix with other linen. Towels for cleaning should not be mixed with the linen for packing, at any time.

All the articles in the theater should be used with importance of its own and never misused. Once it is used, it should be cleaned and replaced. Trays, basins and other utensils need more attention in this connection. Arrangement and order should be insisted always. Lending and borrowing articles between theater and ward should be avoided. Anything which is given to the ward in unavoidable circumstances should not be brought inside without sterilization, e.g. airways, Ryles tube, catheters, IV drip connections, forceps, screwclip or drainage tube, etc.

When patients are brought to the theater for operation they are received in the premedication room, and immediately before they are shifted to the theater trolley from the ward trolley, their dress is changed with the theater cloth and vice versa after operation. Trolleys, wheeled in the floor of the ward should not be allowed to roll in the floor of the theater other than the premedication and recovery room. Ward trolleys should not be allowed to wait in any of these rooms. Remember that the floor of the ward is not like the theater and ward linen and blankets should be used in ward trolley and theater linen should be used in the theater trolley.

Observe the principles in the cleaning, sterilizing and the use of instruments and needles for operation and its after care. Special care should be taken in the case of delicate and sharp instruments. Remnants of absorbable suture materials should be discarded as we have no means of proper sterilization of the same. Non-absorbable materials should be sterilized again by autoclaving if there is balance which is not contaminated during operation. Outside of the glass tubes containing the suture materials should be sterilized according to the instructions given on the packing boxes by the suppliers, before they are taken to the sterile trolley.

Strictly follow the principles in preparation, preservation and utilization of sterile materials. Gloves and other rubber articles used for dirty operation should not be used for clean cases as rubber articles are not satisfactorily sterilized like metal instruments after contamination. Special attention is taken in the preparation of gloves, patched or old gloves should not be prepared for major operation. During operation, surgeon, assistant and scrubbing nurse should change their gloves before opening the peritoneum as they all have touched on the external parts for the procedure before the skin towel is put.

Central sterilization supply is preferred but materials from the theater should not be autoclaved along with the articles from the general ward. Stick on to the principles while packing materials in the drums or bundles for autoclaving. Even though the use of the signaloc is a reliable source of checking the effectiveness of autoclaving, bacteriological test should be practiced to assure the efficiency of the autoclave at least once in a week. If possible sterilization of instruments by boiling should be replaced by autoclaving. When boiling method is used, the sister should supervise the procedure and follow the principles properly.

Specimens, after operation should be kept in airtight containers, immersed in formalin and preserved in a separate cupboard in separate room till they are sent to the pathology department. Prevent foul smell and decomposition of tissues while it is in the theater. Waste materials are disposed properly.

Do not allow to harbor dust or any other dirt material at any part of the theater. Corners and creases in the cupboard or any furniture should be cleaned and the Sister should be alert in supervising the cleaning process. Maintain a scrupulously clean surface everywhere. Dry wiping is never allowed. Always practice wet wiping. Use separate cleaning materials for the articles in the main operation room and other rooms. Wet cloth used for wiping the operation table, instrument trolleys, Boyle's machine, Mayo stand, etc. should not be mixed with cloths using to clean the walls or floor.

Have enough number of all categories of workers for the efficient and systematic work of the theater. Specialized nurses should be allowed to take the responsibilities and to work in the special branches of surgery such as neurology, cardiac surgery, etc.

Advice, encourage and recommend more nurse's and technicians to specialize in operation room techniques and other special branches of surgery and to work in the unit.

Non-technical staff should be given proper instructions while they are posted in the theater and avoid very frequent change of duty for them, whenever possible incidental teaching should be given to them by the nurses. They should be supervised properly to prevent any contamination or complications occurring due to their ignorance. Newcomers should be oriented properly, it is sometimes noted that surgeons, other doctors and other male workers carelessly smoking in the corridors of the theater. This should not only polute the atmosphere of the theater but also cause danger due to fire where the inflammable drugs, gases, etc. are kept in. This behavior should be strictly prohibited. Theater Sister has full power to check any such malpractices within the boundary of the theater unit.

There will be occasions in which instruments and other materials for operations are to be given outside the hospital for family planning camps, eye camps. etc. In such cases balance of perishable articles like cotton, thread, etc. should not be received back to the theater but used in OPD or medical wards. Valuable things like instruments and drums should be received back only after intermittent sterilization.

Nurses should be assigned to particular rooms and definite work should be allotted to other workers so that each one will feel more responsible about their works. This duty should be changed in rotation at few months intervals so that all will become familiar with the functions and no work will be pending in the absence of one or two members. Specialized nurses in particular branch of surgery should be given preference to such particular operation rooms. The theater sister should do a close supervision in every rooms.

Along with the practice of these mentioned measures, a good, theater nurse will do a continuous study of the postoperative period of the daily operated patients in the ward. This should help to note the standard and effectiveness of aseptic techniques in the operation room. The data collected in this matter should be evaluated and discussed with other nurses in the operation room to make necessary alterations and improvements in the functioning. Also, such matters should be brought to the Head of the Department of Hospital such as Surgeon, Nursing Superintendents and Administrators during the Administrative Board meeting. This will help the surgeons to remind their role in the matters and to establish a better co-operation in maintaining the discipline of the theater. There must be discussion and decisions about the actual situation, drawbacks and the required changes for preventing the contaminations and maintaining a high standard of aseptic techniques in the theater for the betterment of the individual patients, successful surgery and increasing the prestige of the institution.

8 Setting up of Instruments

GENERAL SET OF INSTRUMENTS

A collection of generally useful instruments including knives, scissors, hemostasis, dissecting instruments, tissue forceps and retractors is commonly referred to as the 'general' or 'laparotomy' set.

In the following sections, where lists of instruments for various operations are given, the complete lists are set up in some instances: in others only the special instruments that are needed in addition to the general set only mentioned.

The general set used in the hospital in which these were compiled is listed below:
1. Sponge-holding forceps-4
2. Towel clips-6
3. a. No. 4 knife with No. 20 blade and No. 3 knife handle with No. 10, 11 or 15 blade
   b. Mayo scissors straight 1 pair and curved one pair
4. Toothed dissecting forceps, short-2
5. McIndoe's curved dissecting forceps-2
6. Non-toothed dissecting forceps, short and long each
7. One dozen curved fine hemostats
8. One dozen 6-inch Spencer Well's artery forceps
9. Two Moynihan's gallbladder clamps
10. Two large Langenbèck's retractors
11. Two Mathew's retractors

12. Kelly's deep retractors-2
13. Suction nozzle, tubing and quiver
14. Sponge-holder for deep mopping-2
15. Four Doyen's and two Backhaus's tetra clips
16. Two Doyen's intestinal occlusion clamps
17. Two Allis's and two Littlewood's tissue forceps
18. One pair of scissors for the surgeon's assistant
19. Mayo-Hegar needle-holder
20. Suture scissors, ligatures and sutures.

Ligatures

- Thread, size 90 or 60
- Serum-proofed black silk, 3/0 or 2/0 USP (United States Pharmacopocia)
- Catgut, plain-size 2/0 or 'o' chronic, size 1 or 1/0
- Sutures and needles
- Intestinals sutures, chromic catgut 2/0 on small curved atraumatic needles
- Peritoneal sutures, chromic catgut 1/0 or 1 on curved round-bodied needles
- Muscle and fascia sutures, chromic catgut 1 or black silk 2/0 or 1/0 on curved round-bodied needles
- Subcutaneous sutures, plain catgut 2/0 or 1/0 on curved round-bodied needles.

Skin sutures, silk 2/0 or 3/0 or nylon 5N in cutting needles. Michel's skin clips with rack and applicator. Tension sutures are sometimes used: silk 1 or 1/0, nylon 8N (extra stout) or braided nylon 12 lbs on large curved cutting needles. The tension sutures are threaded through half-inch lengths of capillary rubber tubing to prevent the sutures from cutting through the skin.

Abscess Incision (Opening an Abscess)

1. Sponge holding forceps-2
2. A Bard Parker knife handle (No. 3) and No. 10 blade 1
3. Two pairs of long non-toothed dissecting forceps

Setting up of Instruments 65

4. One pair of surgeon's sharp-pointed scissors, one pair of suture cutting scissors
5. A long curved cutting-edged needle
6. Thread for securing the rubber drain
7. Corrugated rubber drain, rubber tube and safetypin
8. One pair of toothed dissecting forceps
9. A culture tube and swab
10. One pair of sinus forceps
11. Probe
12. Two pairs of Kelly's hemostat forceps.

Amputations

For amputations through the arm or leg a selection from the following instruments will be required in addition to the general instruments except large retractors. Amputations of fingers and toes are often carried out by disarticulation through a joint. The nurse should ascertain beforehand the site of the operation and the surgeon's wishes with regard to the type of saw and bone instruments to be set and prepared.

1. Gigli wire saw, handles and De Martel's guide
2. Wood's jaw saw
3. Finger saw
4. Metacarpal saw
5. Horsley's skull saw
6. Medium amputation saw
7. Tubby's bone file
8. Faraboeuf's straight rugine
9. Faraboeuf's curved rugine
10. Small amputation knife
11. Large scalpel
12. Large amputation knife
13. Large curved Spencer Well's artery forceps or gallbladder clamps (two usually required)
14. Chisel
15. Mallet
16. Amputation shield for thigh

17. Tourniquet
18. Esmarch's rubber bandage
19. Lane's bone-holding forceps
20. Lane's patella-holding forceps
21. Ferguson's lion bone-holding forceps
22. Metal rule and skin marking
23. Bone-nibbling forceps
24. Bone-cutting forceps
25. Geouge forceps
26. Osteotome.

Operations on the Breast

a. Opening of a breast abscess
   Same as that of opening an abscess. Plenty of gauze rolls are required to plug the cavity.
b. Simple amputation of the breast or removal of an adenoma:
   General set of instruments except large retractors are enough.
c. Radical mastectomy for malignant disease:
   General set of instruments with the addition of:
   Lanes tissue forceps 7"—4
   Diathermy may be used
   Skin grafting may be required.

Appendectomy

Instruments same as for general set.

Bone Grafting

Example Tibia to spine
General instruments: With the addition of the following:
- Cheatle's forceps for handling instruments
- Lane's bone-holding forceps
- Periosteal elevators
- Faraboeuf's rugines
- Bone-cutting forceps
- Bone Nibbling forceps
- Sequestrum forceps

- Sharp spoons
- Hammer, chisels and gouges
- Metal rule
- Albee's or other electrically driven saw
- Drills
- Bradawl
- Screws and screw-holder.

Ball syringes and normal saline solution for irrigating the field of operation. Plaster bandages may be used. The instruments may be set up on two trolleys, one set for taking the graft and the second set for applying it.

Other Bone Operations

Wiring, plating and screwing of fractures, e.g. femur, tibia, patella, ulna.

General set with the addition of the following:
- Instruments except retractors
- Patella-holding forceps
- Lane's bone-holding forceps
- Tubby's bone file
- Screw driver
- Awl
- Two Langenbeck's bone hooks
- Langenbeck's periosteal elevator
- Two Hey Grove's bone-holding forceps with interlocking bar
- Lane's elevator
- Lane's spike
- Faraboeuf's straight rugine
- Faraboeuf's curved rugine
- Chisel
- Mallet
- Wire twister
- Wilms' bone forceps
- Wire cutters
- Small metal calipers
- Screw and plates

- Screw holder
- Osteotome
- Drill handle and drills
- Trotter's bone nibbling forceps
- Wire
- Pliers
- Metal rule
- Drills and screws
- Plate holder and two plate benders.

NB: Screws and plates must be made of the same metal to prevent electrolytic action. Details given previously under the heading metal on page 33.

Bronchoscopy

1. De Vilbiss spray for local anesthetic
2. Non-toothed dissecting forceps
3. Round-ended scissors
4. Lack's tongue depressor
5. Six towel clips
6. Glass measure containing local anesthetic, e.g. amethocaine 2 percent
7. Tall jar containing hot water for telescopes
8. Beacker for lubricant
9. 20 ml record syringe for aspiration
10. Test tube for specimen
11. Small bronchoscope mops in bundles of ten on a safetypin
12. Mop-holder
13. a. and b. telescope
14. Suction tube with elastic gum terminal
15. Light carrier
16. Jackson's bronchoscope
17. Biopsy forceps
18. Long Punch forceps
19. Amethocaine spray
20. Light cable

A laryngoscope may be needed.
If a general anesthetic is used a gag should be provided.

Cesarean Section (Lower Segment Operation)

For this operation the instruments for abdominal hysterectomy will be required in addition to the following:
1. Two pairs of Willett's scalp forceps long
2. One pair of Willett's scalp forceps, short
3. Four green-Armytage's lower segment forceps
4. Wrigely's obstetric forceps
5. Suction tubing and special nozzle
6. Suction tubing and mucus extracting nozzle for the baby
7. Ampoules containing pitutrin, ergometrine and lobeline
8. Syringe and needles for injection of drugs.

Cauterization

Electric diathermy is used.
Instruments required depends upon the area to be cauterized.

Cholecystectomy

The instruments required in addition to the general set:
1. Long straight scissors 8-inches
2. Mayo's curved scissors 8-inches
3. Moynihan's gallbladder forceps, six required
4. Long straight Spencer Well's artery forceps. 8-inch four pairs required
5. Gallstone scoop.
6. Doyen's curved intestinal clamp, two.
7. Doyen's straight intestinal clamp, two.
8. Trocar and cannula
9. Lithotomy forceps
10. Thompson-Walker's stone forceps
11. Desjardin's fenestrated stone forceps
12. Jaque's rubber catheter, size 8 or 10
13. Fine rubber tubing for draining the common bile duct. T-tube may be used and must be tested for potency on the operation table itself.
14. Elastic gum bougies, sizes 5 to 16, for exploring the bile duct
15. 10 ml syringe and exploring needle

16. Malleable probe-ended scoop
17. Flexible probe
18. Suction connection and nozzle
19. Extra tissue forceps. In addition to those on the general set may be needed.

Circumcision

- Sponge holding forceps-1
- Scalpel or Bard-Parker knife
- Two pairs of scissors
- Two fine dissecting forceps, toothed and non-toothed
- Six fine artery forceps
- Sinus forceps
- Prob
- Bone-cutting forceps
- Fine curved triangular needles
- Catgut 3/0
- Dressing of liquid paraffin gauze or tincture of benzoin

Colostomy

Instruments as for gastrectomy will be needed with the following additions:
- Glass or nylon colostomy rod and fixation tube. Three sizes of Paul's angled colostomy tubes
- Two lengths of Paul's latex tubing, wide and narrow
- For cecostomy, a Jacque's catheter size 12 English gauge will be needed.

Colporrhaphy

Colporrhaphy, perineorrhaphy, plastic operations on the cervix, i.e. trachelorrhaphy and amputations of the cervix, vaginal hysterectomy and vulvectomy.

Instruments as for dilation of the cervix, and uterine curettage with the addition of:
- Two dozen hemostats, four pairs of Allis's tissue forceps, a self-retaining catheter, e.g. Foley's may be required.

OPERATIONS ON THE GENITOURINARY TRACT

Cystoscopy, Ureteric Catheterization and Retrograde Pyelography

- A mackintosh, towels and towel clips
- A bowl containing gauze and wool mops
- A large gallipot containing lotion for cleaning the genitalia, e.g. Milton 1 in 160 or Bradosol 1 in 2000 solution. Two large kidney dishes, one containing sterile catheter.
- Lubricant in small bowl
- A set of Clutton's sounds
- A Riches's cystoscope (boilable) in a perforated metal box. The contents of the box are:
- An examining and operating sheath, obturator, examining telescope, single and double catheterizing telescopes, irrigating attachments, light lead
- A bladder syringe
- A small gallipot containing colored surgical spirit for cleaning cystoscope lens. Spirit must be used sparingly or the cement may be damaged
- Ureteric catheters, fine dissecting forceps, syringe, needles adaptor and glass measure. All these sterile articles are set up on a sterile towel
- Culture tubes for catheter specimens from each renal pelvis.

Cleft Palate Repair

- Mouth gag, e.g. Lane's spring gag, Kliner-Dott gag
- Boyle Devis mouth gag
- Tongue clip
- Tongue depressor, cheek retractors
- Fine scalpels, six towel clips
- Six fine artery forceps
- Two fine toothed dissecting forceps
- Two fine non-toothed dissecting forceps
- Two pairs of fine tissue forceps, e.g. Allis's
- Cleft palate scissors or fine pointed scissors
- Cleft palate elevators hooks and raspatories

- Howarth's raspatory
- Suction connection and fine nozzle
- Fine rubber tubing for threading on tension sutures
- Fine triangular needles and special cleft palate needles
- Needle-holder
- Atraumatic sutures
- Plain and chromic catgut size 3/0 and 2/0
- Thread size 60
- A harelip bow may be used
- Fine osteotomes, chisels and a hammer
- All widths of ribbon gauze should be available
- White head's varnish for palate packs
- A strong thread is stitched through the tongue and left *in situ* for the nurse to control the position of the tongue until the patient is conscious
- Good lighting is essential for these operations.

Dental Extraction

- Mouth gag
- Tongue clip
- Dental conveying forceps
- Dental elevators
- Fine scalpels
- Suction apparatus
- Mouth probes
- Tongue depressor
- Set of dental extraction forceps
- Dental probes
- Fine sutures
- Suture cutting scissors-1 pair
- Needle holder 1.

Dilatation and Curettage

- Sponge-holding forceps for preparation of vulva.
- Towel clips
    - Sim's vaginal speculum
    - Lateral wall vaginal speculum

- Two sizes of blades of Auvard's weighted speculum
- Two vulsella forceps
- Silver probe
- Uterine sound
- Set of needle holder, 1 needle holder, Hegar's cervical dilators
- Sharp and blunt uterine curettes
- Sponge-holders or ovum forceps
- Silver and rubber catheters in a sterile kidney tray
- Specimen bottle or test tubes
- Uterine packing forceps.

NB:
- Needle-holder scissors and sutures
- Toothed and non-toothed dissecting forceps, knife and a pair of long curved scissors
- These instruments are required for cervical biopsy.

Excision Jaw

Excision or partial excision of jaw.
- General instruments except large retractors
- Mouth gag, e.g. Waugh's or Ferguson's gag
- Cheek retractors
- Tongue clip
- Tongue depressor
- Small saw, e.g. wood's and circular saw
- Gigli's wire saw, handles and De Martel's guide
- Periosteal elevators, Faraboeuf's rugine
- Bone-holding forceps (Ferguson's lion forceps)
- Large and small bone-cutting forceps
- Small and medium sized osteotomes and hammer
- Drills
- Silver wire
- Pliers
- Bradawl
- Wire cutters
- Suction connection and nozzle
- Tracheostomy may be performed and more rarely gastrostomy also may be done.

Gastrectomy

The general set of instruments with the following additions:
- Jacque's or self-retaining catheter, about size 12 English gauge or size, 20 French gauge, and catheter introducer.
- A small funnel to fit the catheter
- A jug of warm sterile water
- A local anesthetic may be used.

Gastroenterostomy, Partial Gastrectomy and Gastroenterostomy

The general set of instruments with the following additions:
- Diathermy
- Nelson's scissors curved-on flat
- Three dozen fine hemostats
- Two dozen 6-inch Spencer Well's hemostats
- Six gallbladder clamps
- Two Doyen's straight intestinal clamps
- Two Doyen's curved intestinal clamps
- Two Parke-Kerr's intestinal clamps with caps
- One Lane's gastroenterostomy clamp
- Two medium Payr's crushing clamps
- Two deep abdominal retractors
- Atraumatic chromic catgut 2/0 to close the duodenum and make the anastomosis
- Gastric suction apparatus for the anesthetist's use.

The Theater Sister or Nurse responsible must be prepared to discard any equipment soiled by intestinal contents and to supply fresh gowns and gloves for all members of the team. Fresh instruments will also be needed to complete the closure of the wound.

Some surgeons do not consider that this is necessary in surgery of the stomach and small intestine, but it is deemed essential if the unprepared colon is opened.

Laparotomy

Same as general set of instruments.

Hemorrhoidectomy

- Sigmoidoscope may be needed
- Rectal speculum, Kelly's or bi-valve
- Bard-Parker knife or scalpel
- Two pairs of toothed dissecting forceps
- Two non-toothed dissecting forceps
- Scissors, round ended, curved and straight
- One dozen Spencer-Well's artery forceps
- Six towel clips, Sponge-holding forceps
- Six pile clamps or Kocher's clamp forceps
- Needle-holder
- Curved round bodied and triangular needles
- Stout thread, catgut and strong silk to ligate piles
- 2/0 plain catgut to ligate vessels.
- Stout rubber tube, or Pauls latex tube
- Pile injection syringe and needles
- Injection solution (Phenol in almond oil).

Herniotomy

Operation for the repair of hernia.
The general set of instruments will be required with the addition of the following:

- Symond's No. 6 round-bodied fish-hook needles and Gallie's small living fascia needles
- If the fascia lata of the thigh is to be used, it is usually taken subcutaneously and a Rowland's fascia stripper and fascia forceps will be needed.
- If a full-length incision is made in the thigh, sutures of chromic catgut No. 1 should be provided.
- Sometimes plantaris muscle tendon is taken with tendon stripper passed subcutaneously.

Hydrocele

Excision of hydrocele sac.
General set of instruments except big retractors and the following:
- Small retractors

- Tapping the collection of fluid is carried out by means of a hydrocele trocar and cannula.

Operations on Uterus and Fallopian Tubes

Abdominal hysterectomy, oophorectomy, salpingectomy, myomectomy. Operations for shortening the round ligaments and for ruptured ectopic gestation.

The general set of instruments will be required with the following additions:
- Diathermy
- Self-retaining abdominal retractor
- Doyen's pelvic retractor
- Additional sponge-holding forceps
- Nelson's long curved scissors
- Four gallbladder clamps
- Two vulsella forceps
- A myomectomy screw
- A Mayo's needle for stitching the vagina
- Catheters.

NB: A ruptured ectopic gestation requires an emergency operation. The patient is likely to have a considerable degree of shock with bleeding into the pelvic cavity. Plenty of warm abdominal packs should be available and no small swabs which are likely to be overlooked should be put in.

Intestinal Resection

Instruments required same as that of gastrectomy.

Insertion of Radium

Interstitial application of radium:
(for cancer of the tongue)
- Mouth gag, tongue clip, tongue depressor
- Knife handle and small blade
- Six towel clips
- Scissors, round-ended and pointed

Setting up of Instruments

- Toothed and non-toothed dissecting forceps
- Radium needles
- Radium-holding forceps
- Radium rams for pushing the needles into the tissue
- Stout exploring needle to bore holes for the radium needles
- Round needle and long thread stitch to pass through the tongue
- Needle-holder, thread and small triangular needles
- Two-inch roll of gauze for use as a pack
- Sponge-holding forceps
- Suction apparatus with tube and nozzle
- Tracheostomy instruments should be in readiness

When interstitial radium is used in other sites the requirement in addition to the special radium instruments will be those appropriate to the particular method of approach. In most cases general dissecting instruments, a stout exploring needle, and a tenotomy knife will be needed.

Laminectomy

- Special pointed knife for opening dura mater
- Two knives
- Toothed and non-toothed dissecting forceps
- Round-ended scissors
- Small pointed scissors
- Mayo's curved scissors, 8-inch
- One dozen curved Spencer Well's artery forceps
- One dozen straight, Spencer Well's artery forceps
- Faraboeuf's rugines, straight and curved
- Semb's raspatory
- Horsley's seekar
- Sargent's dura mater elevator
- Silver spatula
- Watson-Cheyne's dissector
- Three small hooks
- Balance's double-ended spoon
- Straight Kocher's forceps
- Two Czerny's retractors

- Two Trotter's self retaining retractors
- Mallet
- Gouze
- Chisel
- 20-ml record syringe and fine catheter
- Key's bone-cutting forceps
- Horsley's laminectomy forceps
- Czerny's nibbling forceps
- Trotter's nibbling forceps
- Diathermy needle and lead
- Sponge-holding forceps
- Suction connection and angled nozzle
- Ball syringe in measure containing normal saline
- Gallipot containing Horsely's wax
- Metzenbaum's needle-holders and curved needles
- One with black silk and one with "serum-proof" silk
- Straight skin needles with black silk
- "Patties" of fluffed wool with black threads attached.
- Roll of 1-inch ribbon gauze and strips of lintin.

Lumbar Ganglionectomy

Division of secondary root of:
- Gasserian ganglion
- Skin needles for marking
- Bard-Parker knives
- Two toothed and two non-toothed dissecting forceps
- Scissors, Mayos and Wheeler's
- One dozen curved and one dozen straight artery forceps
- Self-retaining mastoid retractors
- Rake retractors
- Adson's periosteal elevator
- Faraboeuf's rugines, straight and curved
- Brace and burrs
- Rongeur forceps
- Small bone-nibbling forceps, e.g. Wilms'
- Macdonald's raspatory
- Watson-Cheyne's dissector

- Brain spatula
- Sterile match-sticks for arresting bleeding from the middle meningeal artery
- Two small blunt-ended hooks ⎫ Dental hooks
- One sall sharp-ended hooks   ⎭ may be used
- Long tenotomy knife
- Straight skin needles and sutures
- Lintin strips and wool patties
- Corrugated rubber drainage tube and safetypin
- Ball syringe and sterile normal saline solution
- Diathermy: Suction nozzle and connection.

Nephrectomy

Operations on the kidney and ureters, nephrotomy, nephrolithotomy, nephrectomy, nephrostomy and ureterolithotomy

For these operations general instruments with the addition of those shown below will be required. For nephrostomy a self-retaining catheter should be included:

- Two Faraboeuf's rugines curved and straight
- Two Doyen's raspatories right and left
- Key's bone cutting forceps (or rib shears)
- Trotter's rongeur forceps
- Ferguson's lion bone-holding forceps
- Gallbladder forceps, six
- Long Spencer Well's artery forceps, four
- Renal pedicle clamps, two
- Round-ended scissors, 20 cm—1
- Curved Mayo's scissors, 20 cm—1
- Pointed Mayo's scissors, 20 cm—1
- Lithotomy forceps—2
- Thompson: Walker's stone forceps—1
- Deep abdominal retractor—2
- Suction connection and nozzle
- Fine bougies (sizes 5 to 10) for exploring ureters, 10 ml syringe and fine rubber catheter, size 4 to 6
- Two ureteric catheters.

Esophagoscopy

De Vilbiss spray with local anesthetic, e.g. amethocaine 2%
- Non-toothed dissecting forceps
- Lack's tongue depressors
- Round-ended scissors
- Six towel clips
- Glass measure containing amethocaine
- Tall jar containing hot water for telescopes
- Beaker with lubricant, e.g. tragacanth compound
- 20 ml syringe for flushing suction tubes
- Small mops in bundles of ten on a safetypin
- Test tube for specimen
- Mop-holder
- Two suction tubes
- Coin catcher, a pair of rotating grasping forceps may be used
- Dental plate cutter
- Grasping forceps for foreign bodies
- Crocodile forceps
- Punch forceps
- Irwin Moore's esophagoscope and handle
- Negus's esophagoscope
- Amethocaine spray on rest
- Light cable
- If a general anesthetic is given a mouth gag should be provided
- Litmus paper should also be available.

Oophorectomy

Read operations on uterus and fallopian tubes on page 76.

Perineorrhaphy

Read colporrhaphy on page 71.

Suprapubic Prostatectomy

- Mayo's curved scissors 20 cm—1
- Mayo's pointed scissors 20 cm—1

- Round-ended scissors, 20 cm—1
- Two Skivington's tissue forceps (straight vulsellum forceps may be used)
- Long Spencer Well's artery forceps, four
- Moynihan's gallbladder forceps, six
- Harris's boomerang needle
- Harris's suture-holding forceps
- Harris's retractor
- Lithotomy scoop
- Lithotomy forceps
- Anterior blade of Thompson-Walker's retractor
- Thompson-Walker's self retaining bladder retractor
- Suction connection and nozzle
- Marion's suprapubic drainage tube (a piece of stout rubber tubing or a self-retaining catheter may be used)
- Jaque's rubber catheter, size 12 or 14
- Elastic gum catheter, size 21 French gauge
- Wooden spigot
- Catheter lubricant
- Bladder syringe.

Proctoscopy

- A battery and leads
- A proctoscope with light and leads
- Non-toothed dissecting forceps used as a mop conveyor with proctoscope
- Bellows with lens
- Biopsy forceps
- A bottle with label for biopsy specimen
- A metal suction nozzle with rubber tip
- Crocodile mop carriers
- Large sigmoidoscope sheath with obturator
- A dressing mackintosh and towel
- Mops and lubricant
- Gauze and cotton mops small enough to pass through the sheath of the sigmoidoscope

- A bowl containing water to clear the suction tube
- Suction apparatus
- If the patient is conscious the sigmoidoscope should be warmed.

Skin Grafting

- Magill's suction nozzle
- Skin-marking pen
- McIndoe's non-toothed dissecting forceps
- 12 cm straight sharp-pointed scissors
- McIndoe's scissors
- Kilner's skin hook
- Gillies' skin hook
- Catspaw retractor
- Bodenham Humby's skin graft knife and guard, with disposable blades
- Metal measure, skin graft board, fine sutures in fine (eye) curved cutting needles, fine needle holders
- Plenty of sterile normal saline.

Suprapubic Cystostomy

General set of instruments with the following additions:
- Diathermy, Thompson Walker's bladder retractor
- Selection of self-retaining catheters, e.g. Malicot's or De Pezzer's catheters and introducer
- Drainage tubing
- Bladder syringe
- Warm solution for irrigation
- A trolley should be prepared for cystoscopy and bladder "fill-up"
- Cystostomy may be performed through a suprapubic stab wound using a bladder trocar and cannula.

Thyroidectomy

Operations on the thyroid gland.

The general set (with the exception of Kelley's retractors and Doyen's intestinal clamps) will be required:

- Two dozen curved hemostats
- Self-retaining thyroid retractor
- Thyroid enucleator
- Jame's Macdonald's blunt dissector
- Syme's aneurysm needle
- To medium-sized Langenbeck's retractors
- Two small Langenbeck's retractors
- Diathermy point, handle and lead
- Small drainage tubing, latex or Dunhill's and a small safetypin may be required
- Michele's clips on rack with forceps
- Ligatures and sutures, plain catgut 3/0 and 2/0' or silk 3/0 and 2/0 USP
- Fine cutting needles
- If a bandage is used, it must be light and loose.

When moving the patient the head must be carefully supported to preserve the sutures in the platysma muscle.

Additional instruments which will be required for operations for a thyroglossal cyst or sinus or for a retrosternal thyroid gland are:
- Small periosteal rugine
- Bone-cutting forceps
- Sternum splitter or osteotome and hammer.

Urethrotomy

External Urethrotomy (Wheelhouse's Operation)

- Knife
- Non-toothed dissecting forceps, 12.5 cm
- Non-toothed dissecting forceps, 17.5 cm
- Round-ended scissors
- One dozen Spencer Well's artery forceps
- Wheelhouse's staff
- Lister's steel sounds (a full set should be provided)
- Probe-pointed director
- Teale's gorget

84 Operating Room Technique and Anesthesia

- Jaque's rubber catheter, size 10 or 12
- Harris's drainage tube
- Roll of 2.5 cm ribbon gauze
- Wooden spigot
- Tape for tying catheter
- Bladder syringe
- Nylon sutures and curved triangular needles
- Spool of catgut
- Needle-holder, round-bodied needle and catgut
- Six towel clips
- Catheter lubricant
- 1:1000 solution of flavine.

Internal urethrotomy

- Silver catheters
- Benique's sounds
- Urethrotomy knives
- Filiform bougies, the end screw on to the guide marked
- Grooved guide for urethrotomy knives
- Elastic gum catheter size 21 French gauze
- Malecto's self-retaining catheter, size 18
- Catheter introducer
- Wooden spigot
- Tape (this may be used for tying in a urethral catheters)
- Bladder syringe
- Catheter lubricant.

Examination for Patency of the Fallopian Tubes

- Gas insufflation
- Vaginal bayonet retractor
- Vaginal speculum, e.g. self retaining or Sim's duckbill
- Four towel clips
- Two Vulsella forceps
- Uterine sound
- Hegar's dilators, small sizes
- Measure containing water at a temperature of 105°F

- The intrauterine nozzle of the gas insufflation apparatus and the connecting tubing must be sterilized
- A stethoscope should be provided.

Salpingography

- Injection of iodized oil, followed by X-ray examination
- Sponge forceps
- Vaginal retractor
- Vaginal speculum
- Four towel clips
- Two Vulsella forceps
- Special syringe for oil and intrauterine nozzle, e.g. Fosdyke's to fit syringe
- Container of iodized oil standing in a bowl of warm water.

Vesicovaginal Fistula: Repair of

- Instruments required for colporrhaphy plus
- VVF knife, VVF scissors
- Mosquito forceps-12
- Long non-toothed dissecting forceps-2
- VVF sponge holder (Fine-2)

VVF needle cutting and round-bodied, serveral with black silk or No. 000 atraumatic catgut 3 tubes, sterile gention violet or methyline blue solution. Ounce glass, 20 cc glass syringe and extra kidney trays.

Vasectomy

5 cc syringe, suitable hypodermic needles, drugs for the local anesthesia and a small cup for the drug

- Sponge holding forceps-2
- Towel clips-2 to 4
- BP handle and blades
- Scissors-2 pairs
- Artery forceps-2
- Alleys tissue forceps-2

- Skin needle-1
- Round bodied curved needle-1 or an aneurysm needle
- Needle holder-1
- Silk and cotton thread
- Fine catgut
- Required dressings

A thick pad of cotton is needed to place under the scrotum, while bandaging after operation.

Bandage long enough to support the scrotum.

(Some surgeons use two additional hypodermic needles for lifting the vas before incising the skin).

Postpartum Sterilization (PPS)

- Towel clips-4
- Sponge holding forceps-2
- Alley's tissue forceps-2
- BP blades with handles-2
- Spencer Well's artery forceps-6
- Mayo's scissors-2
- Suture cutting scissors-2
- Toothed dissecting forceps-1
- Non-toothed dissecting forceps-1
- Needle holder-1
- Mathew's retractors small-2

Needles

- Round bodied half circle curved needles-2
- Fascia needle-1
- Skin needle straight-1
- Catgut plain No. 1
- Catgut chromic No.1 and cotton thread for the skin.

ENT OPERATIONS

Mastoidectomy

- Myringotome
- Two scalpels

Setting up of Instruments 87

- Curved bistoury
- Toothed and non-toothed dissecting forceps
- Scissors, round-ended 20 cm-1
- Pointed scissors 15 cm-1
- One dozen fine curved hemostats
- Keen's angular forceps
- Tilley's angular forceps
- Faraboeuf's rugine
- Freer's dissector
- Probe
- Two Dundas-Grant's probes
- Single hooks (blunt and sharp)
- Two double hooks
- Two double-ended retractors
- Tongue clip
- Mollison self-retaining mastoid retractor
- Lack's tongue depressor
- Mason's gag
- Magnifying glass
- Suction tubing and aural nozzle
- Curved artery forceps
- Balance's spoon
- Volkmann's spoon
- Heath's mastoid hammer
- Chisels
- Gouges
- Fine-toothed and non-toothed dissecting Forceps 17.5 cm
- Ribbon gauze and fingerstall plugs
- Gallipot containing adrenaline 1:1000
- Silk worm gut, catgut, thread and triangular needles
- Needle-holder with curved needle
- Sponge-holding forceps
- Ligature forceps
- Four towel clips
- Gruber's aural specula, small, medium and large.

Polypectomy, Intranasal Ethmoidectomy and Removal of Nasal Polyp

- Tongue clip
- Tongue depressor, Mason type gag
- Sponge-holding forceps
- Four towel clips
- Thudicum's and two Kilian's expanding nasal specula
- Postnasal sponge and introducer
- Tilley's dressing forceps
- Luc's forces
- Dissector, Freer's or Hill's
- Straight probe
- Dan Mackenzie's polypus forceps
- Punch forceps, e.g. Grunwald's ethmoid forceps and Hartman's nasal punch
- Ethmoid curette
- Scissors
- Two snares
- Suction nozzle and connection.

Tonsillectomy (Tonsillectomy and Curettage of Adenoids)

- Two towel clips
- Mouth gag
- Tongue depressor
- Tongue clip
- Long, fine toothed dissecting forceps
- Boyle-Davis's gag with large and small tongue depressors
- Mollison's pillar retractor
- Tonsil dissector
- Long, fine dissecting scissors
- Tonsil snare
- Three curved Sidney Scott's 20 cm, artery forceps
- Two long, straight, artery forceps, 20 or 25 cm
- Fine catgut or thread ligatures and scissors
- Adenoid curettes
- Mackenzie's tonsil needle
- Long, non-toothed dissecting forceps

- Luc's forceps
- Sponge-holding forceps
- Suction tubing with pharyngeal nozzle
- Fine suction catheter with graduated connection for postnasal space.

Tracheostomy

- Sponge-holding forceps
- Four towel clips
- Range of needles for local anesthetics
- 10 ml syringe
- Glass measure for local anesthetic
- Scalpel for the skin
- Tenotome-type scalpel
- Short toothed dissecting forceps
- Fine curved hemostats
- One short and one long pair of non-toothed dissecting forceps
- Six fine curved hemostats
- Small self-retaining retractor
- Two double hooks, blunt-ended
- Ligatures, fine thread size 90 or fine silk 3/0 USP or plain catgut 3/0
- Sutures: silk 3/0 USP or plain catgut 3/0 on small half curved cutting needles
- Skin sutures, silk 3/0 USP or nylon 5N on fine straight or curved cutting needles
- Scissors
- Mayo-Hegar needle holder
- Scissors for surgeon's assistant
- Two pairs Allis's tissue forceps
- One sharp hook
- Durham's pilot and outer tracheostomy tube
- Two inner tracheostomy tubes-Durham's
- Tracheal dilators
- Catheter and graduated connection for suction through the inner tube
- Metal suction nozzle
- Thick-walled suction tubing and quiver for suction nozzle.

EYE OPERATIONS

Cataract Extraction

Record syringe and needle for injection of local anesthetic, e.g. 4 percent, Novocaine
- Wright's needle-holder curved needle and black silk, size 1
- Eye speculum for the right eye and left eye
- Fixation forceps
- Graefe's cataract knife
- Moorfield's curette
- Cystotome and curette
- Dressing forceps
- De Wecker's Iris scissors
- Iris forceps
- Three Iris repositors
- Lens scoop
- Lens scissors
- Lid retractors
- Undine with rubber tube and nozle for second irrigation of anterior chamber
- Gauze dressing
- Gamgee, pad
- Moorfield's bandage
- Undine in triangular tray for first irrigation.

Enucleation of Eye

- Eye speculum
- Fixation forceps
- Scissors
- Dressing forceps
- Squint hook
- Stout curved scissors for division of nerve
- Straight scissors
- Spencer Well's artery forceps
- Wright's needle-holder with curved needle and black silk, size-1
- Eye swabs, dressing and bandage
- Undine in triangular tray for irrigation.

9

Instruments: Specifications and their Uses

In this unit, a list of common instruments, its specifications, and uses are given. Corresponding diagrams are also given. Many of the instruments are named along with the names of its founder which is good in many ways. But the actual name of the instrument is much more important in clinical field, for example, towel clips of different types: When it is needed on the operation table while draping a patient, the surgeon asks for a "towel clip" but not specify the name of the founder, still at times when a particular towel clip is required the surgeon may ask for the particular type. But adding the name of the founder, along with, is an attribute to the person as well as to differentiate the item.

NAMES OF GENERAL INSTRUMENTS

Rampley's Sponge-holding Forceps (Fig. 9.1)

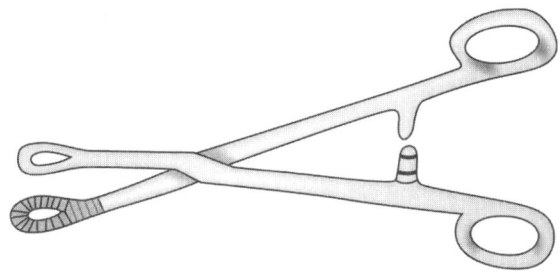

Fig. 9.1: Rampley's sponge-holding forceps

Specifications

1. It is a heavy metal instrument 23-75 cm in length
2. Shafts are thin, blades are fenestrated at it's distal end
3. The inner aspects of the blades are serrated
4. It has a catch lock which gives firmness while holding anything.

Uses

1. Very common use is for cleaning the operative field
2. For swabbing or packing body cavities like vagina
3. It can be used to catch soft organs of the body like ovary, soft cervix in pregnancy, etc.
4. Used for blunt dissection in deeper area
5. Substituted in the place of ovum forceps
6. Used for deep mopping to clear the area during manipulating works on organs.

Towel Clips (Figs 9.2A and B)

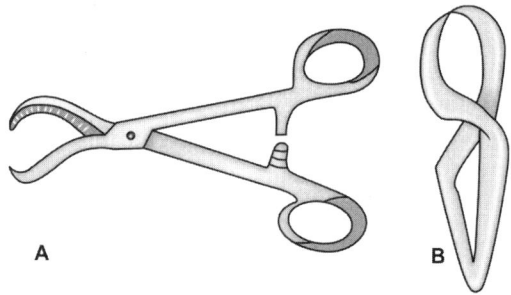

Figs 9.2A and B: (A) Mayo's towel clip and (B) Doyen's towel clip

The common types are:
1. Mayo's towel clip
2. Backhau's towel clip
3. Doyen's towel clip
4. Moynihan's tetra skin clip.

Specifications

1. It is a metal instrument, light but strong, in different lengths
2. It has a catch lock near by the proximal end to fix the grip of drapes
3. The distal ends are curved to two sharp points as teeth, to catch the drapes firmly with the pointed tips
4. Shafts are short and its handles are curved.

Uses

1. To fix the drapes in any manner to expose only the required area
2. To fix the tubings like suction tubes to the drapes preventing displacement
3. To hold or elevate the ribs in chest injuries
4. Can be used as tongue holding forceps, but the disadvantage is that it perforate the tongue
5. It may be used to hold and retract the cord during hernia repairing operation.

Moynihan's Tetra Clip (Fig. 9.3)

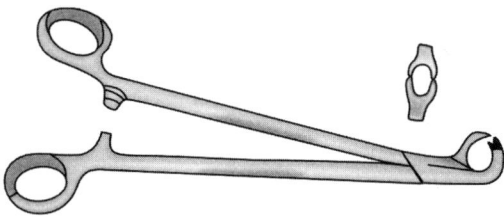

Fig. 9.3: Moynihan's tetra clip

Specifications

It is like any other towel clips. But it has four teeth at the distal end and the shaft is longer than the other clips.

Uses

The important use of tetra clip is to cover the incisional skin edges with sterile drapes all around so that the chances of contamination is reduced. It is used after putting the incision on the skin at any area. It is fixed in position before shifting the fascia over the muscles in abdominal operations.

Bard Parker Knife Handle (BP Handle and Blades) (Figs 9.4A to C)

Specifications

1. It is a metal instrument used to attach different types of blades at the distal end
2. Shaft is flat with 1 cm, breadth at the middle

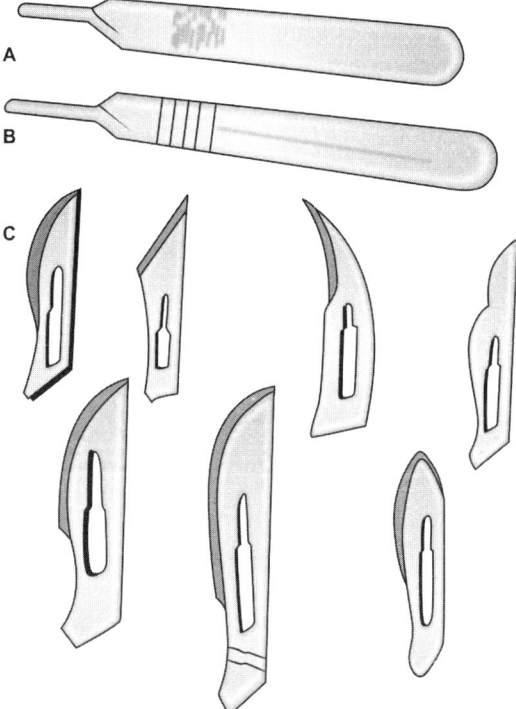

Figs 9.4A to C: Bard Parker handles and blades: (A and B) Bard Parker knife handles, and (C) Blades of different types for the BP handles

3. The distal end is narrow enough to fix the blades with an adjustment to fit on the handle
4. The proximal flat end is round
5. Different sizes of handles are required to fix different sizes of blades according to their uses.

There are scalpel handle combined with blades and scalpel handle with detachable blades.

Uses

1. Scalpel is the most important instrument in surgery
2. Same BP handle can be used for opening the skin and to cut the fascia or to open the peritoneum by changing the blades then and there.
3. The round proximal end of the BP handle may be used to dissect the muscle on the abdomen after cutting the fascia over it.
4. Handing the BP handle and blades may be in the 'dinner knife' position, 'writing position' or in 'Fiddle bow position' while putting the incision.

Scissors (Figs 9.5A to D)

Scissors are of different sizes and designs for the particular uses.
a. Straight scissors (Mayo's) may be blunt or sharp
b. Curved Mayo's scissors
c. Curved on angle (Episiotomy scissors)
d. Curved on flat scissors (Mayo's)
e. Gauze or bandage cutting scissors
f. Stitch cutting scissors may be curved or angled or straight fine pointed tips.

Uses

1. Scissors can be used for blunt or sharp dissection
2. Cutting the tissues in various structures
3. For cutting the ligatures and sutures
4. Gauze or bandage scissors are used only for cutting the gauze or bandages in required size and length.

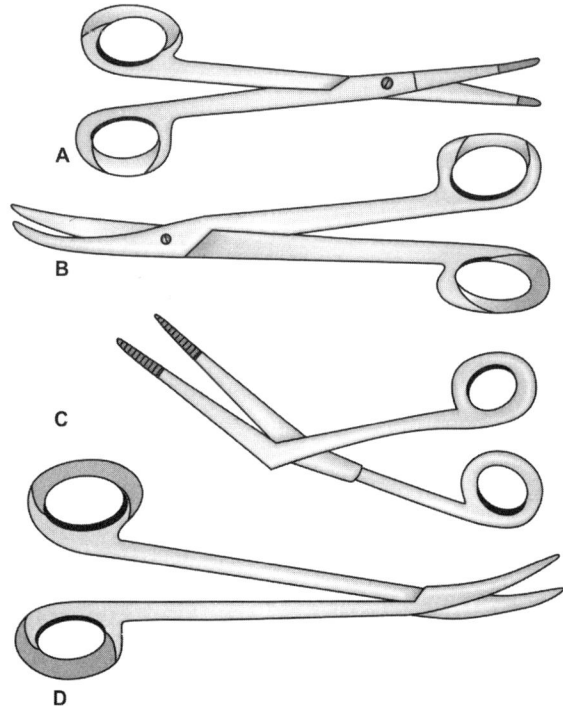

Figs 9.5A to D: Scissors: (A) Straight Mayo scissors, (B) Curved Mayo scissors, (C) Episiotomy scissors, and (D) Suture cutting scissors

5. Straight or pointed curved scissors are used for removing the sutures of the incisions
6. Curved on flat scissors used to cut the ligatures or other suture material during operation by the assistant surgeon or scrubbed nurse.
7. Straight or curved Mayo scissors which are very smooth at the ends used to cut the tissues and internal organs so that adjacent tissues are protected while using.

Dissecting Forceps (Figs 9.6A and B)

It may be non-toothed or toothed dissecting forceps.

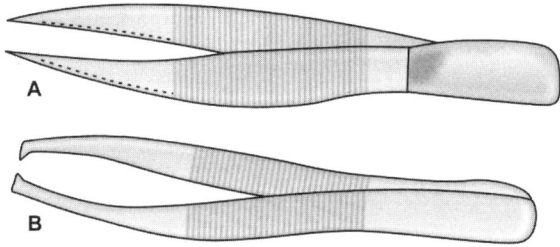

Figs 9.6A and B: Dissecting forceps: (A) Non-toothed dissecting forceps, and (B) Toothed dissecting forceps

Specifications

1. Dissecting forceps has two equal flat wings joining by a sharp curve at the middle which is the proximal end
2. On pressing their shafts or limbs the pointed tips are well apposed so that it do not slip against each other
3. The outer surfaces of the shaft are made rough and irregular to get the firm grip while holding in the hands
4. Toothed dissecting forceps have tooth in the inner surface of the distal end
5. There is a special type of Russian forceps, fenestrated clubbed tip with a serrated inner surface to have firm hold over the soft tissues preventing damage.

Uses

1. Plain dissecting forceps are used to hold the delicate structure like intestine, skin over the face and cartilages for stitching purposes
2. It is used in dissecting soft friable structures
3. Toothed dissecting forceps are used to hold the tough structures like skin, fascia, rectal sheath, etc. while suturing
4. To lift the knots of sutures put on the incision while removing the same after healing the wound
5. Russian forceps are used to hold the skin for suturing or to hold the soft tissues preventing the damage to the organs.

Hemostats (Artery Forceps) (Figs 9.7A to C)

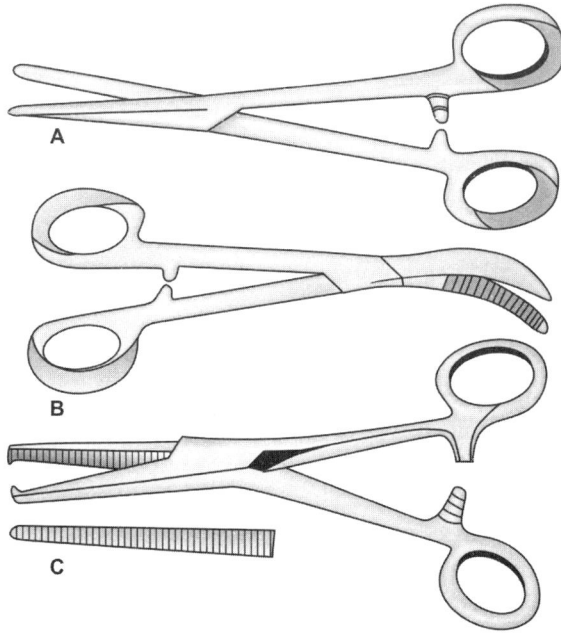

Figs 9.7A to C: Hemostats: (A) Straight artery forceps, (B) Curved artery forceps, and (C) Kocher's forceps

Artery forceps may be:
1. Small or mosquito (straight or curved)
2. Medium
3. Large or pedicular
4. When it is single toothed at distal end it is called Kocher's artery forceps or Lane's artery forceps
5. Non-toothed type may be Spencer Well's or Halstead's artery forceps.

Specifications

1. It is a straight or curved strong metal instrument
2. Blades are tapering to the distal end but blunt
3. It has a catch lock to bring the blades together and lock it

4. The inner surface of the blades are serrated and on locking the blades are well in apposition.

Uses

1. It stops the bleeding on catching the vessel
2. Use as a clamp for the pedicles of internal organs like kidney, spleen, ligaments of uterus, etc.
3. To hold the tip of appendix and crush the base of the appendix
4. To substitute in the absence of sinus forceps to enlarge the opening of an abscess
5. To introduce small plug or drain in a small cavity
6. To substitute in the place of a needle holder
7. To hold the incised edges of skin, fascia, etc. but rarely used due to crushing of tissues.
8. To hold the free end of sutures at the beginning of sutures and hold the cut ends of tension sutures before tying
9. To hold the tape in the abdominal pads or sponges during operations to prevent missing it in the cavity
10. To hold the free end of thread or catgut during anastomosis of intestines
11. Mosquito forceps are used to hold the small bleeding points
12. Used for blunt dissection by holding peanut or swabs.

Kocher's Forceps (Fig. 9.7C)

Uses

1. Kocher's forceps are used to catch the edges of the incision while suturing the skin after operation
2. Used for blunt dissection, holding gauze pallets
3. Specially used to hold the superficial thyroid vessel
4. To hold the ribs in rib resection
5. Used in artificial rupture of membranes in midwifery
6. To hold the retracting vessels in tough fibrous tissues such as in palms, soles and scalp.

RETRACTORS (FIGS 9.8A TO I)

Single Hook Retractor (Fig. 9.8A)

Specifications

It is a flat metal instrument resembles aneurysm needle but no eye at the sharp end. One end is sharp which ends in a hook. The other end is smooth and flat.

Uses

It is used to retract the skin while suturing subcutaneous tissues.

Double Hook Retractor (Fig. 9.8B)

Specifications

It is a multi hooked retractor with two or more pointed edges like cat's paw.

Uses

1. It is used to retract tough structures like fascia of sole and palms
2. The pointed multi hook at the end gives firm retraction.

Doyen's Retractor (Fig. 9.8C)

Specifications

1. It is a heavy metal instrument with a special hook like bent at the tip of the handle
2. The blade is wide and flared in both sides laterally and the tip is well flexed to one side to totally to retract good hold of tissue.

Uses

1. To retract vast area of tissues in pelvic and abdominal operation
2. It can be modified as self retaining refractor by attaching a lead weight to the handle.

Deaver's Retractor (Kelly's Deep Retractor, Fig. 9.8D)

Specifications

1. It is a large metal retractor with broad and slightly curved blade
2. Handle is long and the end is curved like a hook which provides better grip
3. This type is available in various sizes.

Uses

1. It is mainly used in retracting abdominal organs like spleen, liver, etc. The gentle curve prevents much crushing of the organs. An abdominal pack is kept in between the blade of the retractor and vice versa to prevent direct pressure injury to the organ.
2. Smaller retractors of this type can be used to retract bladder walls in intravesical operations
3. In the operations of large intestine or appendix this retractor provides clear visualisation by retracting the pelvic organs and prevent injuries to that organs.

Langenbeck's Retractor (Fig. 9.8E)

Specification

It is a metal instrument with flat solid blade on one end and a long handle. The long handle helps to hold the instrument without obstructing the work of the surgeon. This type of retractor may be seen with blades in both ends but without special handle. It is named Morris' retractor with double blades.

Uses

1. It is used for retracting skin edges or big blood vessels and nerves.
2. It is useful in operations like hernioplasty involving a lot of superficial dissection and retraction of tissues.
3. Morris retractor with double blades is specially used to retract strong structures like abdominal wall and muscles. The beak at the end of the blade gives firm hold over the tissues and the concavity at the blade gives wider area for the work of the surgeon.

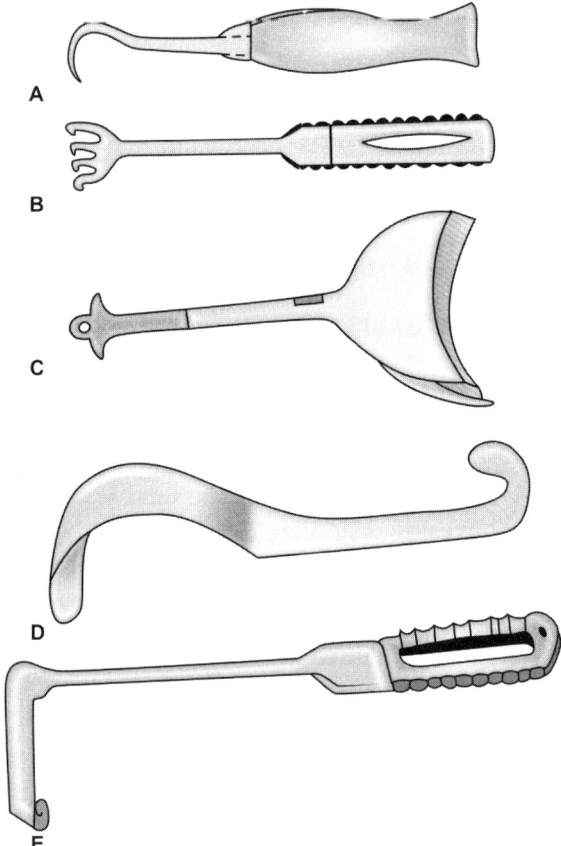

Figs 9.8A to E: Retractors: (A) Single hook retractor. (B) Double hook retractor. (C) Doyen's retractor. (D) Deaver's deep retractor. (E) Langenbeck's retractor

Balfour's Self-retaining Retractor (Fig. 9.8F)

Specifications

1. It is a large metal instrument with special fittings for retaining in the space
2. Rectangle metal pieces are connected together and two small retracting blades are attached to both ends of the rectangle pieces by metal rods. The rods are slightly curved to give space in between

3. There is a middle blade for the retractor which is adjustable by means of screw locks fitted at the middle. This is a detachable blade.

Uses

It is used to retract the organs in abdominal surgery for prolonged time. As it is self retaining the works of the assistant is lessened.

Czerny's Retractor (Fig. 9.8G)

1. It is a metal instrument with fenestrated shaft, not so heavy
2. There is a small and thin blade bent and directed to one side and a double ended hook like blade bent and directed to opposite side.

Uses

1. It is good for superficial retraction of tissues
2. Thin blade is used to retract the margins of any incisions
3. The hooked end is used to retract the ends of incision during the closure of an abdominal wound
4. The hooked end can also be used to retract deep tissues while putting the deep stitches during closure of a wound.

Joll's Thyroid Retractor (Fig. 9.8H)

Specifications

1. It is a metal instrument specially prepared with clip like provisions to hold the incised margins
. It has two flanges which are connected by a metal curve in the middle and a metal adjustable rod is fitted in between the wings of the metal curve
3. The terminal end of the flanges have two clips like sharp teeth on each side which is adjustable at different angles by means of a screw mechanism.

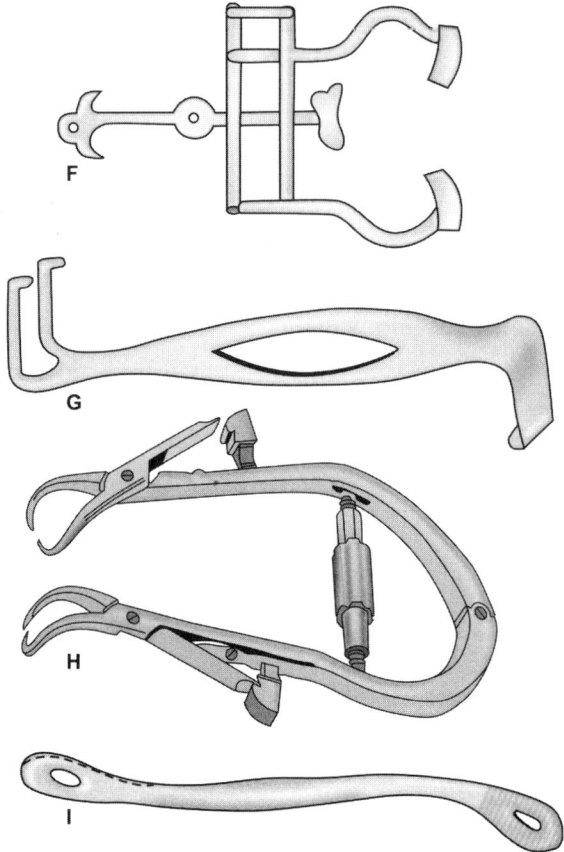

Figs 9.8F to I: Retractors: (F) Balfour's self-retaining retractor. (G) Czerny's retractor. (H) Jolls' thyroid retractor, and (I) Anterior vaginal wall retractor

Uses

1. It is used for self-retaining purpose for thyroid operations
2. It is adjustable to different angles.

Anterior Vaginal Wall Retractor (Fig. 9.8I)

Specifications

1. It is a metal instrument with two oval shaped and fenestrated ends

2. The fenestrated ends have transverse serrations
3. The oval shaped ends are connected at an angle of 45° to both ends of the shaft.

Uses

It is used with Sims' speculum to retract the anterior vaginal wall for exposing the cervix and the anterior fornix.

Suction Nozzle and Tubing (Figs 9.9A and B)

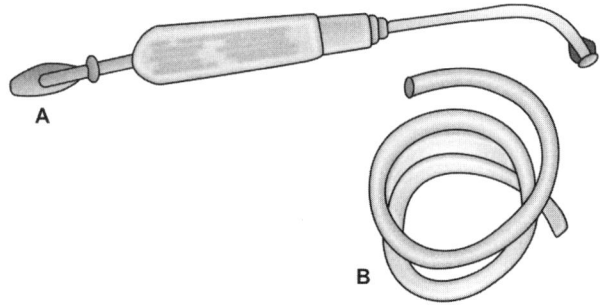

Figs 9.9A and B: (A) Suction nozzle, and (B) Tubings

Specifications

1. Suction nozzle is a metal instrument attached to the distal end of the rubber tubing
2. The proximal end of the rubber tubing is attached to the suction bottle or the reservoir. Usually the suction apparatus is foot operated
3. The distal end of the suction nozzle is protected with perforated tips to prevent the sucking of tissues during functioning or atleast a small rubber tube is fitted at the tip.

Uses

1. It is used to suck off the blood or fluids from the cavities like mouth, abdomen or fluids from a large ovarian cyst, etc. during operations so that the field of operation is cleared.

2. Being metal and rubber it can be sterilized along with other instruments to use in the sterile field. While a vacuum is produced in the suction bottle the fluid or blood is sucked through the nozzle to the rubber tube and collected in the bottle.

Gastric Occlusion Clamp (Fig. 9.10)

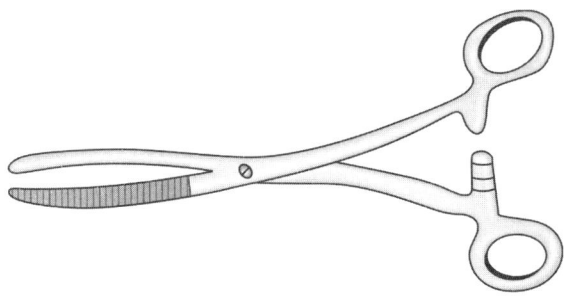

Fig. 9.10: Gastric occlusion clamp

Specifications

1. It has long and strong blades to have a good grip over a great width of stomach
2. The blades are deeply serrated and may be fenestrated so that it gives firm grip and prevents slipping of the walls of the stomach
3. Blades may be straight or slightly curved laterally
4. It is non-crushing occluding clamp.

Uses

It is used to hold and occlude the stomach, during gastrectomy, gastrojejunostomy, etc.

Payr's Gastric Crushing Clamp (Fig. 9.11)

Specifications

1. It is a heavy stout metal instrument
2. The handles have a double lever arrangement with four joints which is the mechanical advantage of this instrument by

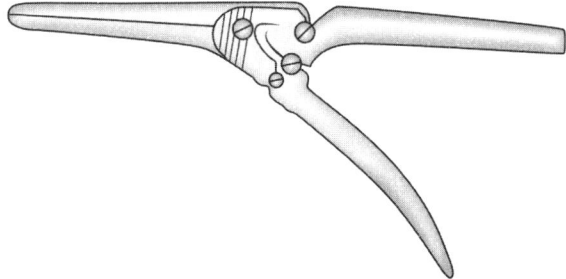

Fig. 9.11: Payr's gastric crushing clamp

increasing the pressure to the maximum effect with limited effort. The instrument has two levers. The first one is for firm apposition of blades and the second lever amplifies the pressure exerted to the handle resulting firm closure without the tendency for the handles to spring apart.

Uses

It is used for partial or total gastrectomy in cases of gastric ulcer, the initial stage of gastric neoplasm, gastrojejunostomic stomal ulcer.

Allis Tissue Forceps (Fig. 9.12)

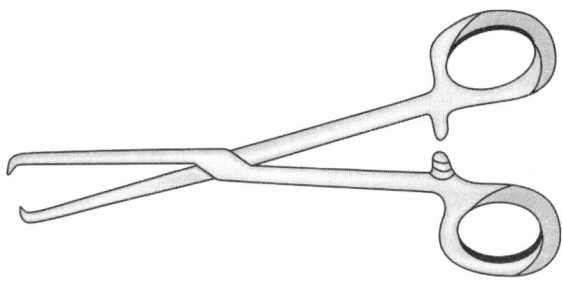

Fig. 9.12: Allis tissue forceps

Specifications

1. It is a metal instrument and its blades are straight along its long axis and are separated by a space except at the tip.

2. There are sharp teeth at the tip which interlock on closing and there is catch-lock mechanism for closing.

Uses

1. It is used to hold thin, but tough structures to give traction on these structures, e.g. for holding skin, fascia, hydrocele sack etc.
2. It can be used to hold tissues with fibrous capsule of an organ for dissection
3. It can be used to hold the bladder neck while doing operations on the neck of the bladder.

Needle Holder (Fig. 9.13)

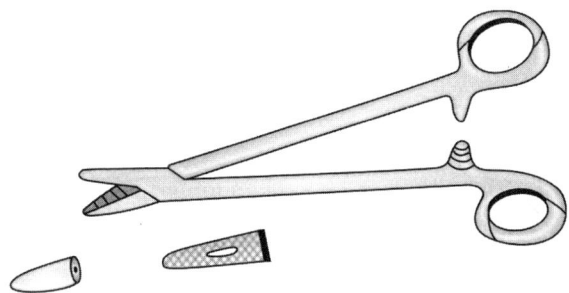

Fig. 9.13: Needle holder

Specifications

1. It has got long handles and small blades resembles artery forceps
2. The blades have very good cross serrations
3. It has a groove for catching the needle on its inner surface
4. It may be straight or curve.

Uses

1. To hold the needle for suturing
2, Straight type is used for holding needles while suturing at surface; curved type is used to work at depth or inside the cavity.

Suture Needles (Figs 9.14A to D)

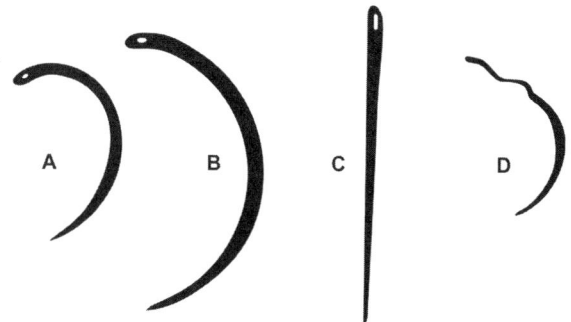

Figs 9.14A to D: Needles: (A) Round bodied. (B) Curved cutting. (C) Straight cutting needle, and (D) Atraumatic

Specifications

1. Suture needles may be specified
   a. On the basis of its edge
   b. On the basis of its curvature
   c. On the basis of its eye
   d. Atraumatic eyeless needles is that the suture material is swaged into the blunt end of the needle so that no injury to the tissues occur due to the doubling of the suture material at the eye end. It can be used only once.

Uses

1. Cutting needle is used for stitching the tough structures like skin and fascia.
2. Round body needles are used for suturing soft and delicate structures.
3. Straight needles are used for giving mattress sutures in the skin.

Aneurysm Needle (Fig. 9.15)

Specifications

1. It is a metal instrument resembling a hook. Tip is blunt which avoid any injury to the surrounding tissues

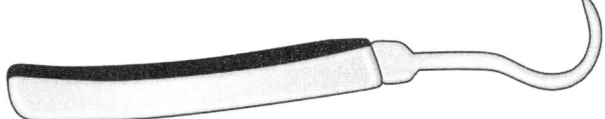

Fig. 9.15: Aneurysm needle

2. There is an eye at the tip and is curved laterally or at right angle to the shaft
3. Eye of the needle is preceded by a groove for the ligatures.

Uses

1. Ligation of aneurysm
2. Ligating vessels in continuity
3. To hook out and ligating a vein during venesection
4. It is used to ligate the cystic duct.

Lister's Sinus Forceps (Fig. 9.16)

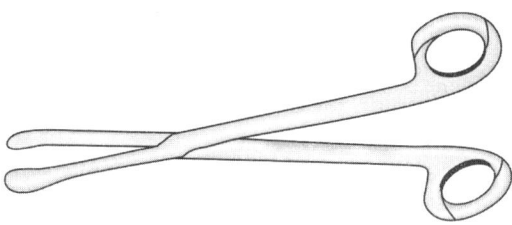

Fig. 9.16: Lister's sinus forceps

Specifications

1. It is a metal instrument with about 24 cm long
2. It has two blades, shaft and handles
3. The distal tip is round blunt and smooth with serrations inside the tip. There is no lock for the grip.

Uses

To introduce rubber drainages or gauze plugs freely in any cavity like ears, nose, cavity of abscess. As there is no lock, the material can be introduced in the cavity without strain and pain to the patient.

Trocar and Cannula (Fig. 9.17)

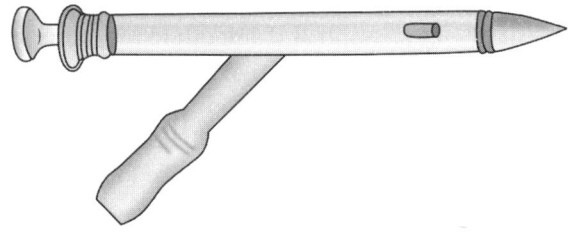

Fig. 9.17: Trocar and cannula

Specifications

1. It is a metal instrument with hollow outer tube and sharp trocar with handle at proximal end
2. The trocar is slightly longer than the cannula and is fitted into it.

Uses

1. It is used to puncture a big ovarian cyst to reduce the size before its final removal. Trocar is pushed in, cyst is punctured and trocar is removed. Then the required amount of fluid is taken from the cyst through the cannula till the size of the cyst is such that it can be removed easily. After the fluid has been removed the wall of the cyst can be closed by Pyesmith's clamp
2. It is also used to puncture the abdominal wall in ascites by paracentesis
3. It can be used to puncture the abdominal wall in cases where laparoscopic operations are intended. Here a laparoscope is introduced into the abdomen through the cannula after removing the trocar.

Probe (Fig. 9.18)

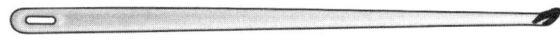

Fig. 9.18: Probe

Specifications

1. It is a very thin and long metal instrument about 24 cm or more in length
2. The distal end is round and smooth to introduce in any cavity smoothly. Usually there is an eye in the proximal end through which a long thread can be introduced, which helps to find out the probe when put in deep cavity. If the probe is fully immersed to the depth of a cavity there is chance for missing it inside. In that case the thread will be seen outside so that the metal probe is located easily.

Uses

1. To introduce in any cavity to note the depth
2. To identify the hole of the cervix in pinhole cervix before introducing the uterine sound or dilator.

Cheatle's Forceps (Fig. 9.19)

Specifications

1. It is a large heavy metal forceps with remarkably curved blades
2. Inside the blades there are large serrations which help to get firm grip while taking instruments, vessels or linen
3. There is no lock.

Uses

1. It can be used to select and pick up sterilized articles like drapes, instruments and vessels or even bottles from sterilized drums or autoclave
2. As it is heavy, long and good with serrations, sterile articles can be safely transferred from one tray to another

Instruments: Specifications and their Uses **113**

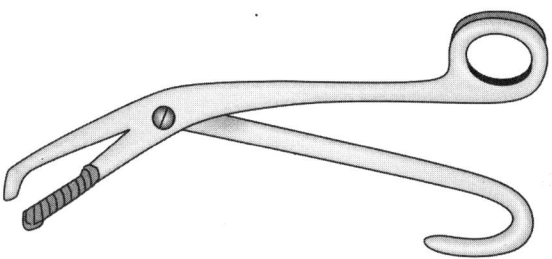

Fig. 9.19: Cheatle's forceps

Usually it is dipped in an antiseptic solution like dettol lotion or carbolic lotion for ready use. It is also called transfer forceps.

Major Abdominal Incisions (Figs 9.20A to I)

Specifications

1. Incisions are made in different size and shape on any part of the body according to the operations to be performed. The major abdominal incisions are:
   Vertical: (a) median—upper or lower, (b) paramedian—upper or lower. Each can be left or right in position
2. Transverse or oblique, e.g. McBurney's incision
3. Alphabetical 's' shaped
   'L' shaped or 'V' shaped
4. Cherney for pelvic exenteration
5. Abdominothoracic incision.

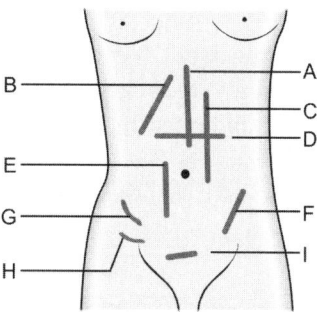

Figs 20A to I: Major abdominal incisions: (A) Midline. (B) Right subcostal. (C) Left upper paramedian. (D) Transverse. (E) Right lower paramedian. (F) Left iliac. (G) Right gridiron. (H) Right lanz, and (I) Suprapubic

Methods of Suturing (Figs 9.21A to C)

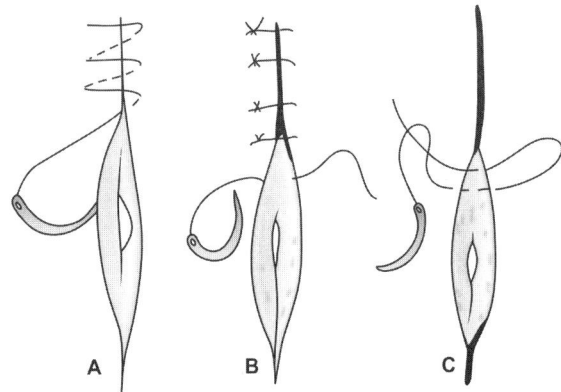

Figs 9.21A to C: Methods of suturing: (A) Continuous suture. (B) Interrupted suture, and (C) Mattress suture

After any planned operation incision may be closed by suturing in different methods depends upon the area of operation and type of incision.

The different types are:
1. Continuous suturing, e.g. closure of peritoneum
2. Interrupted suturing, e.g. skin
3. Blanket or botton-hole suturing, e.g. skin
4. Mattress suturing, e.g. cut muscles and tendons
5. Pursestring suture, e.g. Burying the stump of appendix, burring the cut Fallopian tubes
6. Tension sutures—Tension suture is put about 5 cm laterally away from the original suture of incision to reduce the tension at the incision to prevent gaping the abdomen in very fatty patients
7. Buried subcuticular suturing. It is used where cosmetic importance is more.

SPECULUMS (FIGS 9.22A TO G)

Lang's Universal Eye Speculum (Fig. 9.22A)

Specifications

1. It is a metal instrument designed with two limbs with a spring loaded arrangement
2. These limbs end in a buckled fashion which can be used in right or left eye.

Uses

It is used to retract the eyelids during eye operations, removal of foreign bodies in the eye, cauterisation, etc.

Aural Speculum (Fig. 9.22B)

Specifications

1. It is a metal light weight cone shaped instrument of different sizes
2. In a correctly selected size speculum the tip of it will easily enter the auditory meatus of the patient.

Uses

1. For the examination of the external ear and tympanic membrane
2. It can be used during the operations of the ear if selected promptly
3. To check the extent of damage in the middle ear when the tympanic membrane is destroyed.

Long Bladed Nasal Speculum (Fig. 9.22C)

Specifications

1. It is a light weight metal instrument with two long blades
2. The blades are like two wing's and attached at right angle to a flat metal part joined at the middle which act as the handle.

Uses

1. The blades are brought together before introducing in the nasal cavity and expanded after introduction to the nose
2. It is used to clear the area in nasal surgery.

Killiani's Self-retaining Nasal Speculum (Fig. 9.22D)

Specifications

1. The blades are like any other nasal speculums
2. The handles are the heavy part and it has the self-retaining mechanism.

Uses

1. It is more useful than the long bladed speculum because of its self-retaining action
2. It is used in retracting the tissues in nasal operations.

Auvard's Weighted Vaginal Speculum (Fig. 9.22E)

Specifications

1. It is a weighted vaginal speculum for retaining.
2. The weight is due to the metal weight attached to the handle with suitable curvature to retract the posterior vaginal wall by the blade in operations of the genitourinary system in lithotomy position.

Uses

It is used in operations of the cervix and vagina to retract the posterior vaginal wall.

Sims' Vaginal Speculum (Fig. 9.22F)

Specifications

1. It is a moderately heavy metal instrument
2. It has two thick blades but at both ends laterally to same side

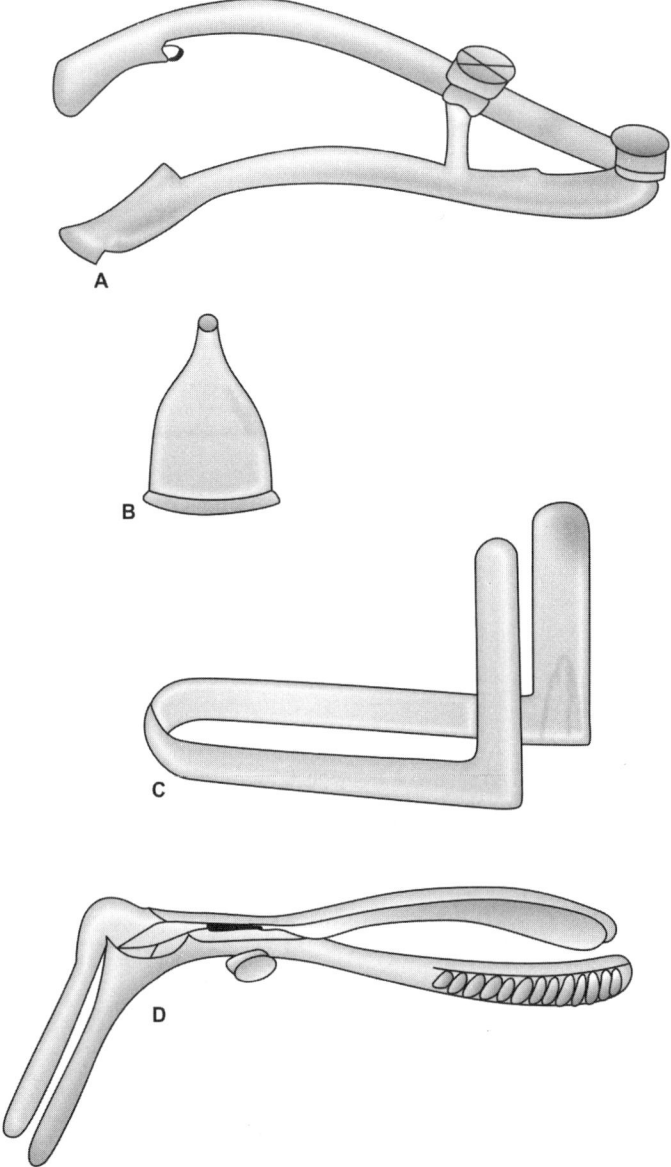

Figs 9.22A to D: Speculums: (A) Lang's universal eye speculum. (B) Aural speculum. (C) Long bladed nasal speculum, and (D) Killian's self-retaining nasal speculum

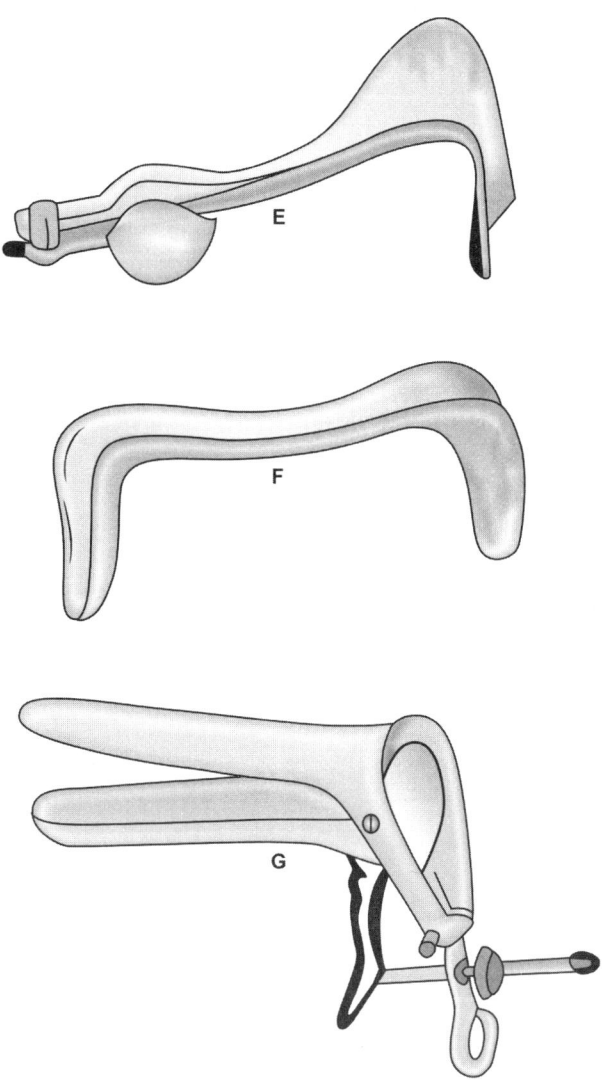

Figs 9.22E to G: Speculums: (E) Auvard's weighted vaginal speculum. (F) Sims' vaginal speculum, and (G) Cus cos bivalved speculum

3. An assistant is needed to hold the speculum in position during operations because it has no self retaining mechanism. It is available in various sizes.

Uses

1. It is used in operations of the cervix and vagina in lithotomy position
2. After placing the patient in lithotomy position with the buttocks at the edge of the bed, one blade of the speculum is introduced along its edge with the blade lying vertically in anteroposterior diameter of the vagina and then rotated to adjust the blade in the vagina. Then the assistant hold at the lower blade and give enough traction downwards according to the required space to be retracted.

Cusco's Bivalved Speculum (Fig. 9.22G)

Specifications

1. It is a self-retaining speculum with a special screw arrangements
2. If has two blades which can be opened laterally and adjusted at various angles by adjusting the screw after introducing in the vagina
3. It is introduced into the vagina with its blades closed in vertical position and made horizontal, opened and locked in positions. It is closed and rotated further and opened up again to see the other sides of the vagina after locking it in the required position.

Uses

1. It is easy to use without any assistance because of the self-retaining action
2. Vaginal wall can be retracted at various angles
3. Every part of the vagina can be visualized by retracting the tissues with the same instrument and it gives good exposure of the cervix

4. It can be used without much discomfort to the patient even without bringing the patient to the edge of the table but the rim of the speculum is an obstruction to limit the space available to carry out any procedure.

GYNECOLOGICAL AND OBSTETRIC INSTRUMENTS (FIGS 9.23A to V)

Simpson's Uterine Sound (Fig. 9.23A)

Specifications

1. It is a light weight metalic staff graduated on the stem
2. It has about 30 cm in length with its distal end is curved slightly at an angle of 60° and about 5 cm in length
3. The tip of the instrument is blunt.

Uses

1. It is used to ascertain the length of the cervix and uterus before any operations of the uterus through vagina
2. It is used as the 1st dilator before introducing the uterine dilators
3. It is used to ascertain the size and direction of the uterus
4. It is used to find out the position of the abnormal uterine contents like tumor, polyp; placental pieces, products of conception, etc.

It is not used in pregnancy or cervical infections. Care should be taken to prevent perforation of the uterus while introducing the uterine sound.

Hegar's Cervical Dilator (Fig. 9.23B)

Specifications

1. Uterine dilators are metal heavy instruments of gradually increasing sizes
2. The marking on the dilators indicate the circumference in millimeters
3. There are various types of uterine dilators like Hawkin's Ambler's cervical dilator, Mathew Dungons dilator, Hegard's dilator, etc.

Uses

1. Dilators are used for dilating the cervix when approach is required through the cervix in pathological conditions of the uterus
2. For dilating the cervix for curetting the uterine contents. Evacuation of the products of conception in MTP or incomplete abortion
3. For insufflation test to note the patency of fallopian tubes
4. In operation of cervix like Fothergill's operation or cauterization of cervix
5. To relieve spasmodic dysmenorrhea
6. For drainage of uterine cavity through cervix
7. For the formation and dilatation of the cervix after cystocele repair operation.

Sims' Double Ended Uterine Curette (Blunt and Sharp) (Fig. 9.23C)

Specifications

1. It is a flat metal instrument with small spoon like arrangement convenient for scraping
2. Both ends are slightly enlarged like small spoon with fenestration in the middle and slightly curved to opposite sides
3. One end is blunt and the other end is sharp for curetting.

Uses

1. To take out the endometrium by curetting the uterine cavity for diagnosis or therapeutic purpose
2. To empty the uterus by curretting the products of conception on incomplete or missed abortion. Complications of uterine curetting are hemorrhage, tears in cervical canal, perforation of uterus and sepsis. Very vigorous curetting may lead to amenorrhea

Flushing Curette (Fig. 9.23D)

Specifications

1. It is a curette with small spoon like arrangement for scraping, at one end.

2. The stem of the curette is hollow for the passage of any fluids to the interior of the spoon like end
3. In the other end a rubber tubing can be adjusted from a reservoir to pass the fluids through the hollow area to the curetting end which is blunt.

Uses

It is used to wash out the uterine cavity by passing fluids through the rubber tube to the curette from a reservoir.

Ovum Forceps (Fig. 9.23E)

Specifications

1. It is a metal moderately heavy forceps having cupped blades with linear fenestrations
2. The size and type of blades can hold a reasonable amount of tissues in between with good grip
3. It is about 30 cm in length.

Uses

1. For removing products of conception from the uterus in case of incomplete or inevitable abortion
2. To remove any foreign body from the uterine cavity
3. To remove any pedunculated polypus from the cervix or uterus by twisting
4. To remove any retained placental or membrane pieces from the uterus after delivery.

Vulsellum Forceps (Fig. 9.23F)

Specifications

1. It is an average size metal instrument resembling a forceps at the proximal end with a lock for fixing. The distal end got sharp teeth which provide firm grip
2. There is a curvature of blades which helps to retract the anterior vaginal wall when the instrument pulled up after holding the cervical lip for better visualization.

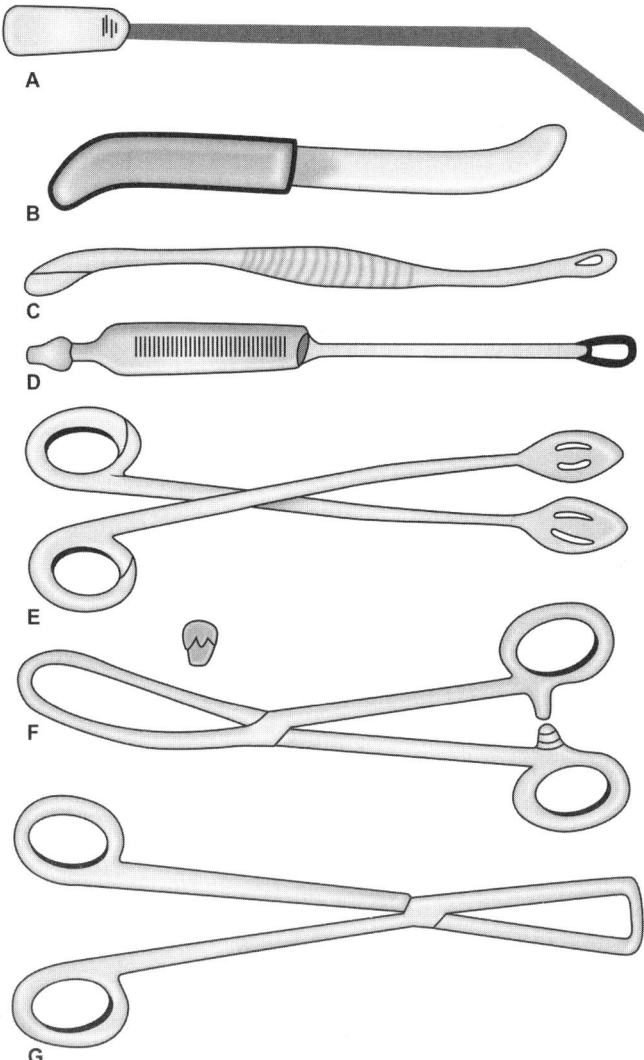

Figs 9.23A to G: Gynecological and obstetrical instruments: (A) Simpson's uterine sound. (B) Hegar's cervical dilator. (C) Sims' double ended uterine curette. (D) Flushing curette. (E) Ovum forceps. (F) Vulsellum forceps. (G) Tenaculum forceps

Uses

1. Used in holding anterior and posterior lip of cervix in various operations like D and C, cauterisation of cervix, etc.
2. To test the mobility of cervix and laxity of ligaments in prolapse of uterus
3. In vaginal hysterectomy it is needed to bring down the fundus of the uterus
4. To hold the cervical lip for procedures like tubal insufflation or introduction of laminaria tent
5. To grasp small fibroids in myomectomy.

Tenaculum Forceps (Fig. 9.23G)

Specifications

It resembles vulsellum forceps except there is single tooth at distal end to hold the tissues of one point only, so that the injury and bleeding is only slight if any.

Uses

It is used to hold the anterior lip of cervix transversely, while doing Rubin's test allows the cannula to fit air tight in cervix and prevent leakage of gas.

Episiotomy Scissors (see Figs 9.5C and 9.23H)

Specifications

It is a type of angle curved scissors with blunt points. There is straight scissors also with blunt points.

Uses

It is used to do the episiotomy in the second stage of labor without causing damage to the surrounding tissues in the perineum.

Green: Armytage Forceps (Fig. 9.23I)

Specifications

1. It is a metal instrument resembling as any other forceps except it has triangular blades with serrated edges.

2. Even when the forceps is fully closed and locked, there is a small space between the blades.

Uses

1. In LSCS it is used to hold the retracted edges of the uterine wall for easy stitching
2. While holding the edges it acts as a hemostat to decrease the bleeding from the incision.

Uterine Packing Forceps (Fig. 9.23J)

Specifications

1. It is a curved forceps about 35 cm in length, curvature corresponding to the axis of birth canal for easy packing.

Uses

1. It can be used instead of laminaria tent applicator
2. Used for vaginal packing to control bleeding from lacerations in the birth canal due to traumatic conditions
3. To pack the uterine cavity in emergencies till medical aid is available
4. To pack the uterus in bleeding when other control measures fail after D and C.

Drew-Smythe Catheter (Membrane Perforator or Cannula) (Fig. 9.23K)

Specifications

It is an 'S' shaped catheter with a blunt stillet.

Uses

1. Used for high rupture of fetal membrane in hydramnios and allow the escape of liquor amnii through it
2. It allows the controlled leakage of liquor amnii
3. It can be passed between the membrane and uterus in some distance before puncturing

4. The high rupture of membrane preserves the dilating effect of bag of waters and reduces the chances of infection and prolapse of the cord.

Polypus Forceps (Fig. 9.23L)

Specifications

It resembles a forceps with grip at the proximal end and a special arrangement to catch the cervical polypus.

Uses

1. It is used to remove the polyp; by catching and turning 2 or 3 times
2. It lessens the chances of bleeding by its firm catching and turning.

Rubins' Tubal Insufflation Cannula (Fig. 9.23M)

Specifications

1. It is a hollow tube, slightly curved with an open end and multiple side holes near the tip
2. A conical distal end behind the tip but around the tube is a special adjustment to press against the external os where the cannula is introduced
3. At the outer end of the cannula, a rubber tubing can be connected for air insufflation from the apparatus.

Uses

1. To test the tubal patency in Rubins' test.
2. To push the radiopaque dye to the inside of the uterine cavity in hysterosalpingography
3. In chromotubation, methylene blue dye is pushed through the tube and spilling of the dye is seen through fimbrial end of fallopian tube by laparoscope.

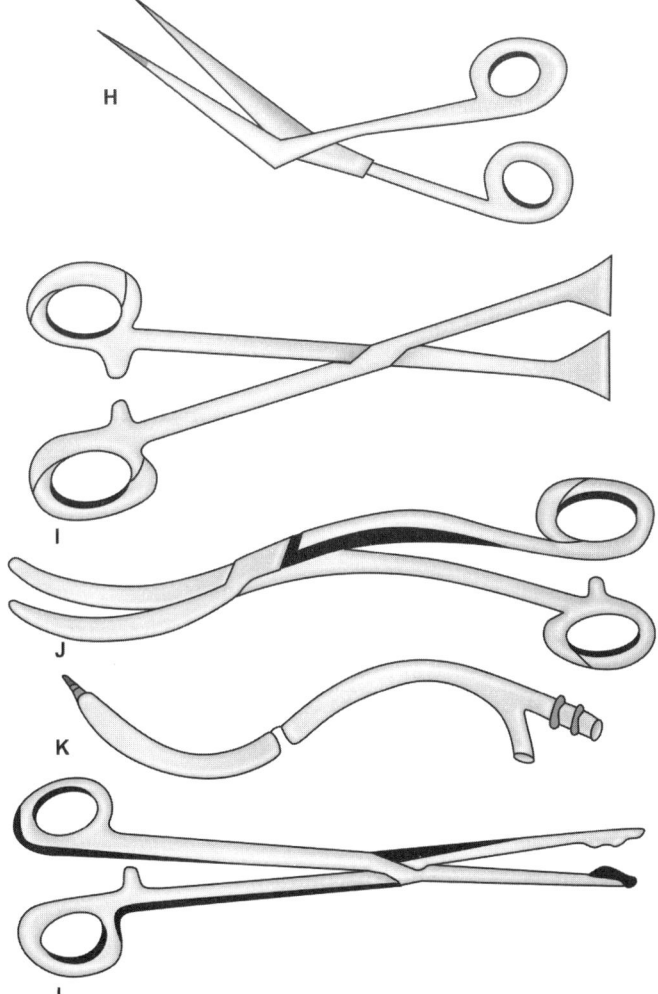

Figs 9.23H to L: Gynecological and obstetrical instruments: (H) Suture cutting scissors. (I) Green Armytage forceps. (J) Uterine packing forceps. (K) Drewsmythe catheter. (L) Polypus forceps

Myoma Hook (Fig. 9.23N)

Specifications

It is a metal instrument in which there is a handle at one end and a sharp hook at the other end.

Use

It is used to hook out the small growths in the layers of uterus.

Hodge's Pessary (Fig. 9.23O)

Specifications

Pessary is a device usually shaped as a ring and is made up of a variety of materials like rubber or plastic. The size and shape of pessary are selected and fitted in the upper vagina of the patient by the gynecologist.

Uses

Pessaries inserted in the upper vagina are positioned to help in keeping the organs such as bladder and uterus is proper alignment.

The patient can be taught to remove the pessary in the night and reinserted in the morning. If it is remaining in place and not removed by the patient she should have it removed, checked and cleaned by a doctor or nurse at prescribed intervals. At this time the tissues need to be inspected for pressure points and irritation. Normally there is no pain, discomfort or discharge with its use. Douching recommended if there is discharge.

Smith's Pessary (Fig. 9.23P)

Specification and uses are as same as Hodge's pessary.

Laminaria Tent Introducing Forceps (Fig. 9.23Q)

Specifications

1. It is a metal instrument with a handle and lock like a forceps, 30 cm in length
2. Blades are slightly bent and concaved at the blunt tip.

Use

To hold and introduce the tent conveniently to the cervix.

Laminaria Tent (Fig. 9.23R)
Specifications

1. It is made up of hygroscopic materials derived from sea weed. It swells up by absorbing fluid causing cervical dilatation
2. It is about 7-10 cm in length like a small pencil with an eye at one end. There is a thread hanging through the eye which is a convenient arrangement while removing the tent.

Uses

1. It is used for dilating the cervix in case of spasmodic dysmenorrhea where the medical treatment is failed.
2. It is used for dilatation of cervix and expulsion of products of conception in MTP, different types of abortion and in hydatidiform mole
3. It is kept in the cervix for 12-24 hrs and by that time the tent becomes swollen by absorbing fluid from the cervix so that os is dilated after the prescribed time.

Carton-Cowell's Mucous Catheter (Fig. 9.23S)

Specifications

It is a metal catheter with special arrangement for sucking the mucus from the throat of the baby.

Willett's Scalp Traction Forceps (Fig. 9.23T)
Specifications

1. It is a forceps with locking mechanism at the handles
2. It has two rectangular obliquely serrated blades
3. Two sharp tiny blades fit into the two holes on the opposite side. The teeth ensures very firm grip on the scalp.

This instrument is not used nowadays as there are better and safer ways of dealing with patients having placenta previa.

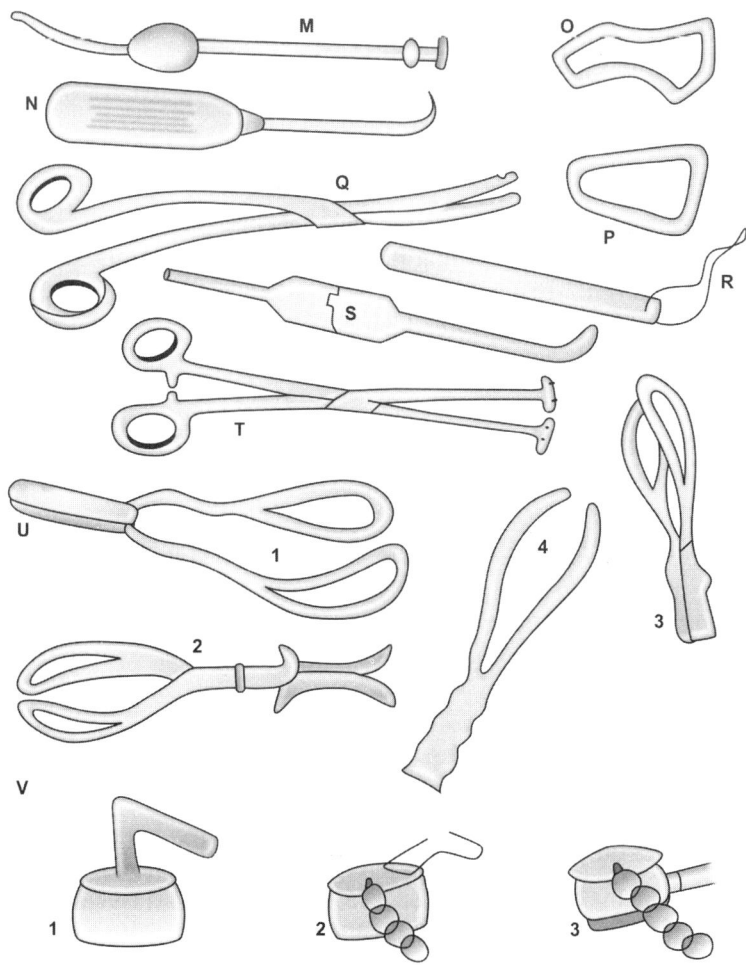

Figs 9.23M to V: Gynecological and obstetrical instruments: (M) Rubins tubal insufflation cannula. (N) Myoma hook. (O) Hodge's pessary. (P) Smyth pessary. (Q) Laminaria tent introducing forceps. (R) Laminaria tent. (S) Carton-Cowells mucuous sucker. (T) Willets scalp traction forceps. (U) 1-4 Obstetrical forceps. (V) 1-3 Vacuum cups

Uses

1. It is used to provide traction over the scalp of the foetal skull presses upon the bleeding site in cases if placenta previa in type I and II in vertex presentation. It is useful only in vertex presentation.
2. Used to pull the head after the cord has been replaced in cases of cord prolapse.
3. Used in cases of cesarean section to disengage the head when required
4. It is used for extracting the fetal head during LSCS and for continuous scalp traction in case of contraction ring obstructing the delivery.

Obstetrical Forceps (Figs 9.23U1-4)

Obstetrical forceps are heavy metal instruments used for extracting the baby in the second stage, i.e. when the cervix is fully dilated. It has two blades, shank and handles. The inner curve of the blade is cephalic curve and the outer curve of the blade is pelvic curve. In axis traction forceps there is a perineal curve also in the traction rods.

Different types of forceps are used to extract fetal head depending upon the descend of fetal head when the cervix is fully dilated.

Vacuum Cups (Figs 9.23V1-3)

Vacuum cups are of different sizes fitting to the tubes of vacuum extractor. Vacuum extractor is an alternative to obstetric forceps in cases where forceps delivery is indicated despite of poor uterine contraction. Traction is applied by this instrument that the cup is made to adhere to fetal skull by creating a negative pressure between vacuum cup and fetal skull.

ANORECTAL INSTRUMENTS (FIGS 9.24A TO C)

Fistula Director (Fig. 9.24A)

Specifications

It is a small thin instrument made up of malleable material. The distal end is blunt and the proximal end has an eye through which thread can be introduced for easy pulling of the instrument out.

Uses

1. It is used to open the fistulous tracts
2. It is used to find out the direction of tracts.

Pile Holding Forceps (Fig. 9.24B)

It is a metal instrument specially designed to hold the inflamed pile in the rectum.

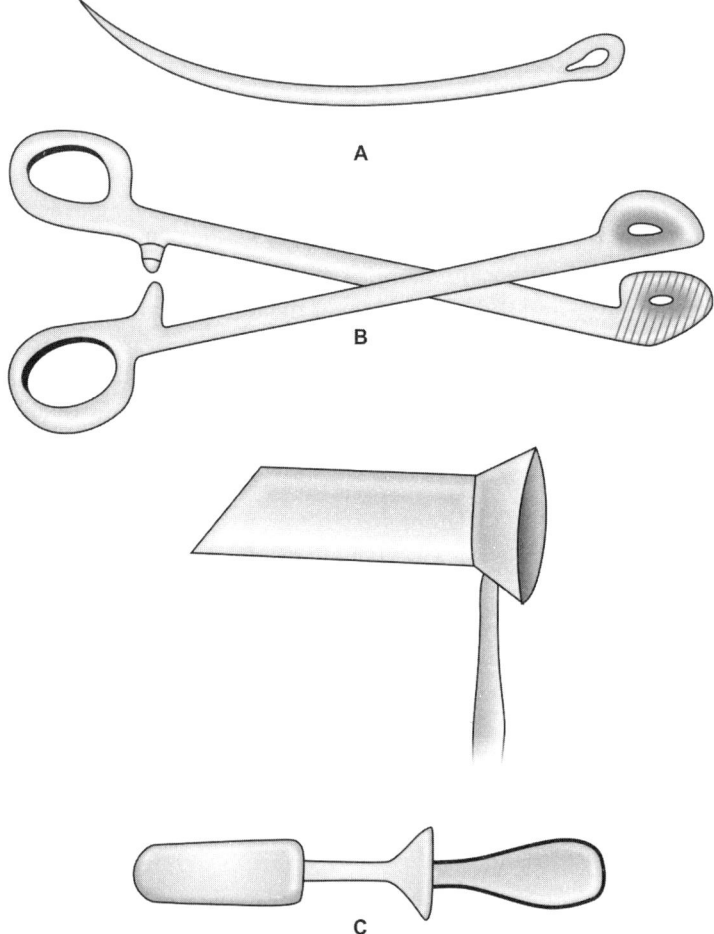

Figs 9.24A to C: Anorectal instruments: (A) Fistula director. (B) Pile holding forceps, and (C) Proctoscope

Proctoscope (Fig. 9.24C)

Specifications

It is an instrument used to visualize the anal canal and the lower end of the rectum. It has two parts, the outer tube and the inner obturator. The outer tube has a handle attached to it. It may have a lighting arrangement inside for the easy visualization.

Uses

1. To find out piles, ulcer or any growth in the rectum
2. It is used in polypectomy, rectal biopsy and pile injection.

EAR, NOSE AND THROAT INSTRUMENTS (FIGS 9.25A to P)

Boyle-Davis Mouth Gag (Fig. 9.25A)

Specifications

This instrument consists of tongue blade attached to a mouth gag which can be opened by a sliding arrangement to retract the jaws. It can be retained in place by attaching its hooked plate to a peg by means of a rope and pulley.

Use

To open the jaws and retract it in oral surgery like tonsillectomy, adenoidectomy, polypectomy, cleft palate, etc.

Crocadile Punch Biopsy Forceps (Fig. 9.25B)

Specifications

It is a forceps with a long slender beak. In the tip of the beak has got two cutting jaws which are manipulated by finger bows.

Uses

It is used to take biopsy through an endoscope like bronchoscope or esopharyngoscope.

Laryngeal Forceps (Fig. 9.25C)

Specifications

It is a long handled curved forceps with a clubbed beak. The beak or tip of the forceps may be cupped with large margins.

Uses

1. To take biopsy from the larynx or base of the tongue
2. To remove foreign body from larynx, pyriform fossa, etc.

Frer's Septal Knife (Fig. 9.25D)

Specifications

1. It is a long slender instrument which has got a sharp knife near its tip.
2. The edge of the knife is directed medially when in use.

Use

It is used to incise the mucosa over the deviated septum.

Luc's Forceps (Fig. 9.25E)

Specification

It is a forceps with bar joint and cutting tip.

Uses

1. This forceps is used in radical antrostomy (Caldwell-Luc operation). Maxillary sinus is opened up through canine approach and the damaged mucosa is stripped off using Luc's forceps. This approach is supplemented by a counter opening in the nasal wall from within the sinus.
2. It is also used for SMR operation for removing the nasal septum (SMR means submucous resection)
3. For taking biopsy from oral cavity and oropharynx
4. Used as a substitute for tonsil holding forceps and for nasal polypectomy.

Denis Browne Tonsil Holding Forceps (Fig. 9.25F)

Specifications

1. It is similar to Luc's forceps in construction except that the fenestrated tip does not have a cutting edge and has simple joint instead of a box joint
2. The long blades are acutely curved on flat so that it does not block the view when in use leaving ample space for using other instruments
3. There is no locking mechanism.

Uses

1. The fenestrated tip allows the bulk of the tissues to bulge out through the fenestration and gives a good grip over the tissues
2. It is used to hold tonsil during dissection and hence its name.

Peritonsillar Abscess Drainage Forceps (Fig. 9.25G)

It is a bayonet shaped forceps used to drain the peritonsillar abscess through an incision given at the junction of an imaginary horizontal line through the base of the uvula and a vertical line along the anterior pillar. The point of incision may be marked by carbolic acid which also acts as an anesthetic and antiseptic.

Eve's Tonsillar Snare (Fig. 9.25H)

Specifications

It is a very powerful snare used in ENT surgery. There is a special arrangement at the proximal end with three circle like metal handle to hold it tightly with three fingers.

Use

It is used to crush and cut the lower polar attachment that is the pedicle of the tonsil.

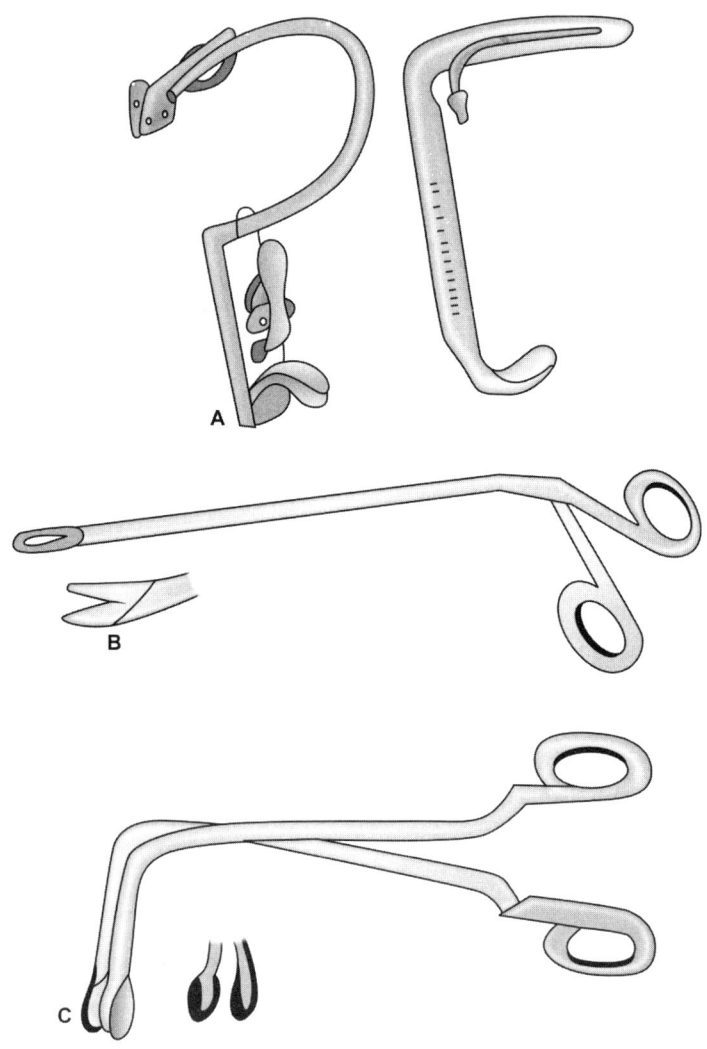

Figs 9.25A to C: Ear, Nose and Throat Instruments: (A) Boyle-Davis Mouth gag. (B) Crocodile punch biopsy forceps. (C) Laryngeal forceps

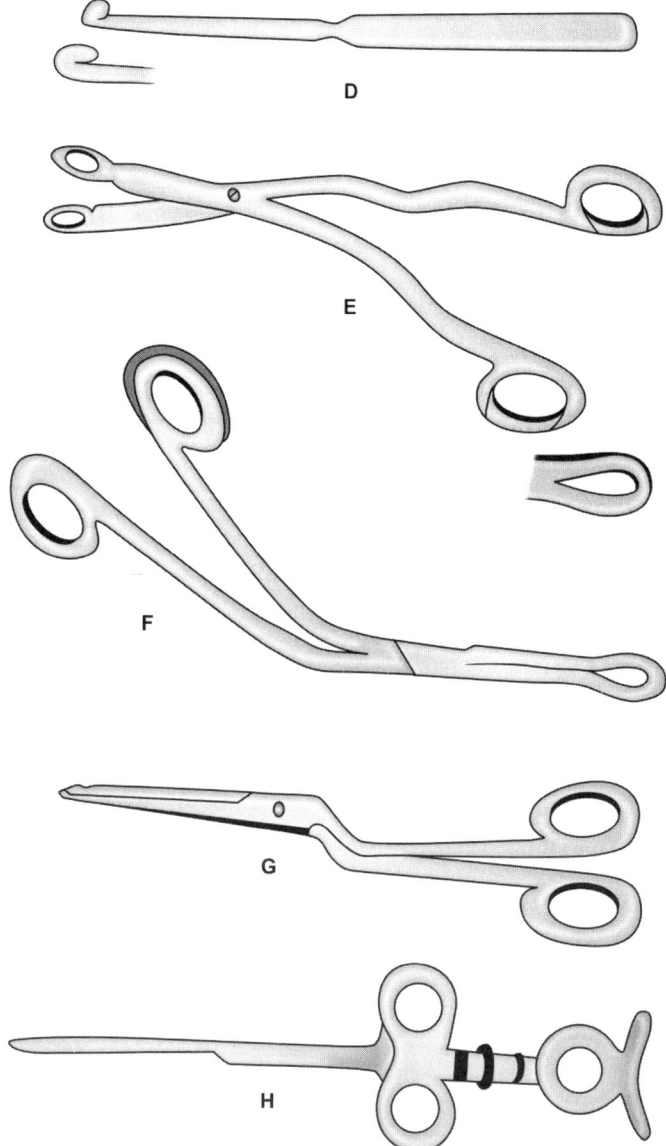

Figs 9.25D to H: Ear, nose and throat instruments: (D) Frer's septal knife. (E) Luc's forceps. (F) Denis Brown tonsil holding forceps. (G) Peritonsillar abscess drainage forceps. (H) Eve's tonsillar snare

Adenoid Curette with Cage (Fig. 9.25I)

Specifications

There are different sizes of curette used to remove even though smaller amount of adenoid tissue is left behind. Handle is large enough to hold in a firm grip. At the distal end the arrangement is sufficient to do the curetting.

Uses

For adenoidectomy this instrument is held as a dagger and is manipulated behind the soft palate. Then it is dagged forward to curette out the adenoids. It is a blunt procedure to start with a large sized curette, but the process is continued. Smaller amount of adenoid tissues left behind.

Tonsillar Dissector and Anterior Pillar Retractor (Fig. 9.25J)

Specifications

It has a sharp dissecting end and blunt retracting end.

Uses

1. The sharp dissecting end is used to drive the mucosa close to the anterior pillar in order to expose the capsule
2. The blunt retracting end is used to follow up the exposed capsule down to the base of the tonsil with minimal trauma
3. It can also be used to retract the anterior pillar to look for any bleeders or any tags of tonsillar tissue left behind the operation.

Mastoid Gouge (Fig. 9.25K)

Specifications and Uses

Used in mastoidectomy operation to explore mastoid antrum and mastoid air cells. It is preferable than chisel because of its concave margin and rounded edge which takes off sleeves of bone very easily. The instrument is held at an acute angle to the surface of bone and the bone is cut from behind towards and from above

downwards directed towards the tympanic antrum. If this instrument is used vertically the following accidents may occur.
1. Fascial nerve and lateral semilunar canal may be in danger anteriorly
2. The lateral sinus may be opened posteriorly
3. Injury to the dura mater and temporal lobe brain may occur superiorly.

Lacks Spatula (Fig. 9.25L)

Specifications

It is a tongue depressor with two parts. A handle and a depressing part. The handle is bent at its lower end to provide a good grip.

Uses

1. It is used for examination of oropharynx. Patient is asked to open his mouth and the anterior 2/3 of tongue is depressed with this spatula. At the same time patient is asked to say 'aa-aa-ah so that soft palate moves up allowing a good view of oropharynx
2. It is used to examine the palatine tonsil and pillars, posterior pharyngeal wall, uvula and soft palate
3. It is also used to depress the tongue during peritonsillar abscess drainage.

Myringotome (Fig. 9.25M)

Specifications and Uses

It is a slender angulated instrument with a short lancet shaped blade at the tip used for incising the tympanic membrane (myringotomy) in case of acute suppurative otitismedia.

In myringotomy a 'J' shaped incision is given in the posterior part of the tympanic membrane after painting the outer ear with antiseptics. The point of the knife should not be passed far enough through the drum as to cause any damage to the middle ear structures.

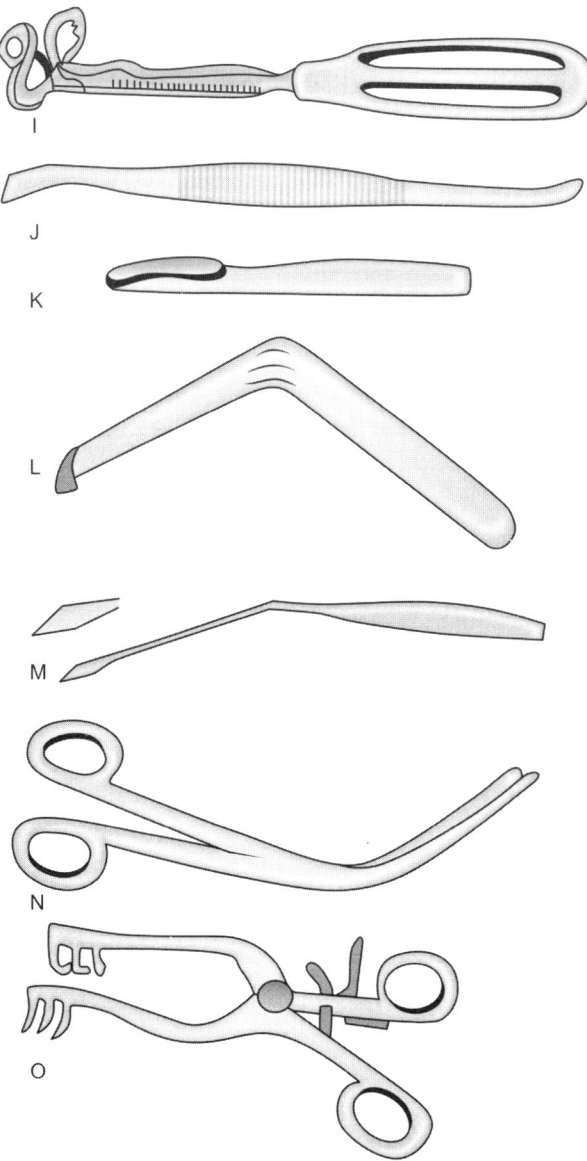

Figs 9.25I to O: Ear, nose and throat instruments: (I) Adenoid curette with cage. (J) Tonsillar dissector and anterior pillar retractor. (K) Mastoid gauge. (L) Lack's spatula. (M) Myringotome. (N) Tilley's nasal dressing forceps. (O) Mastoid retractor

Tilley Nasal Dressing Forceps (Fig. 9.25N)

Specifications

It is a metal instrument with handle and a long blade with blunt tip.

Use

It is used to dress or pack one nasal cavity.

Mastoid Retractor (Fig. 9.25O)

Specifications

It is a self-retaining retractor of hemostatic type available in two sizes. It can be retained in any desired position by its ratchet locks.

Uses

This retractor is used during mastoidectomy operation to retract the skin, subcutaneous tissue and periosteum.

It checks the bleeding from cut vessels in the edges of the incision. Usually two retractors applied at right angles to each other. They are used to open up and retract the postauricular incision margins or exposing the mastoid.

TRACHEOSTOMY INSTRUMENTS (FIGS 9.25P1 TO 6)

Boyle Davis Mouth Gag (Fig. 9.25P1)

Jackson's Tracheostomy Tube (Fig. 9.25P2)

Specifications

It consists of three parts. The inner tube, outer and the obturator. The outer tube has a provision of a lock to inner tube. The tube is fixed in place by means of tapes. The outer tube is introduced along with obturator in tracheostomy. The obturator is removed initially and is replaced by inner tube. Inner tube can be removed whenever, cleaning is required avoiding the need for removal of the tracheostomy tube from trachea. Inner tube is made longer than outer tube so that the latter cannot be obstructed when the inner tube is removed for cleaning.

Modern tracheostomy tubes are made up of plastic and are manufactured with or without an inflated cuff. The cuff is used for mechanical ventilation and needs to be inflated and deflated at regular intervals to prevent pressure necrosis of trachea. Plastic tracheostomy tubes are softer, less irritant, resterilized and disposable.

Chevalier Jackson's Direct Laryngoscope (Fig. 9.25P3)

Specifications

It is an instrument used to observe the larynx. It has got better illumination due to presence of the lighting source just near its distal end. But it has got a slight disadvantage in compromising the internal diameter of the direct laryngoscope.

Uses

1. For detailed examination of hypolarynx and pharynx
2. For removal of foreign body from larynx
3. For taking biopsy from hypopharynx or larynx.

Small Single Hook Retractor (Tracheal Hook) (Fig. 9.25P4)

Specifications

It is resembling BP handle with a hook at the distal end curved laterally. The hook may be sharp or blunt.

Use

It is used to retract skin and platysma muscle in throat.

Trousean's Tracheal Dilating Forceps (Fig. 9.25P5)

Specifications

It is a forceps with bent blades which is blunt at the end.

Instruments: Specifications and their Uses **143**

TRACHEOSTOMY INSTRUMENTS (Figs 9.25P1 to 6)

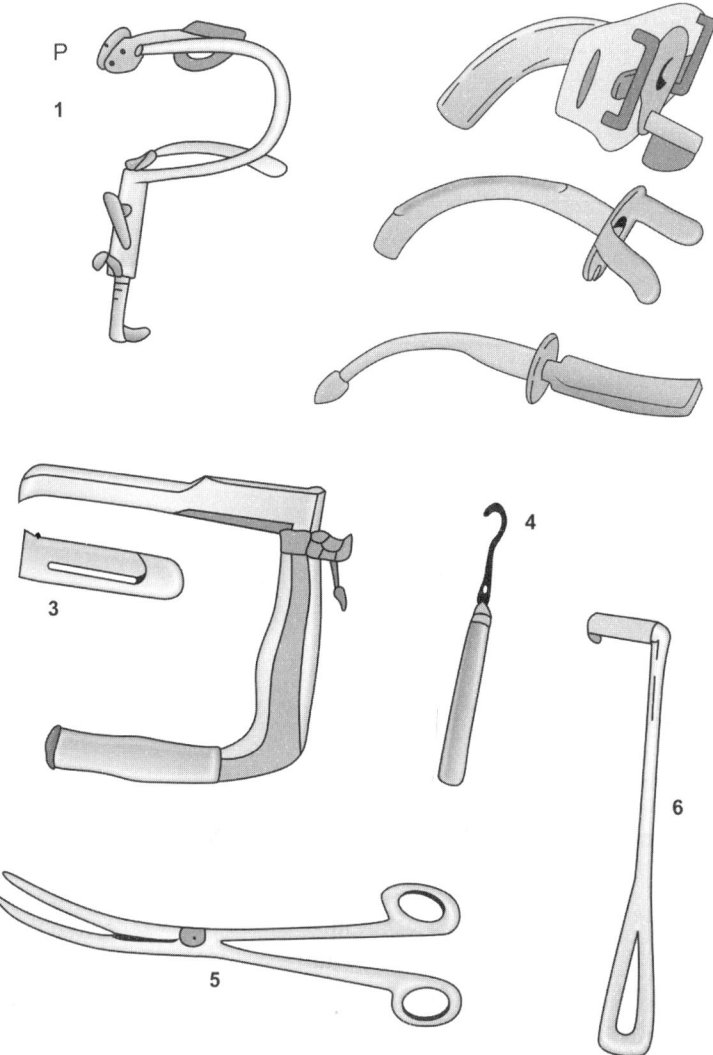

Figs 9.25P1 to P6: Ear, nose and throat instruments: (P) Tracheostomy instruments: (1) Boyle Davis mouth gag. (2) Jackson's tracheostomy outer tube inner tube and piolet or introducer. (3) Chevalier Jackson's direct laryngoscope. (4) Tracheal hook. (5) Trouseau's tracheal dilating forceps, and (6) Langen Beck's retractor

Uses

It is used to dilate the trachea after putting a small incision. That incision is dilated with the forceps to introduce the tracheal tube.

Langenbeck's Retractor (see Figs 9.8E and 9.25P6)

OPHTHALMIC INSTRUMENTS (FIGS 9.26A TO P)

Lang's Universal Eye Speculum (see Figs 9.22A and 9.26A)

Von Graefes Cataract Knife (Fig. 9.26B)

Specifications

It is an instrument with straight blade long narrow and thin with a sharp point and one sharp cutting edge.

Uses

1. For making incision during cataract excision
2. Blunt von Graefes knife may be used for scraping the corneal ulcers
3. In transfixation surgery of glaucoma, iridotomy can be made with this knife.

Straight Needle Holder (Fig. 9.26C)

Specifications

A wide variety of needle holders are available. It has a spring handled limbs and the end of the limb is made finely serrated so that a firm grip over the needle is obtained. They may be available with or without lock.

Uses

For holding the suture needles for fine stitching. It is used in suturing the lids, conjunctival and corneal suturing.

Curette (Fig. 9.26D)

Specifications

It is a long thick needle with a groove in the middle of the broad tip.

Uses

To express out the lens matter during evacuation of congenital cataract or traumatic cataract in children.

Fixation Forceps (Fig. 9.26E)

Specifications

These are stoutly made forceps with two into three teeth at its tip. There are 3:5 or 4:5 toothed forceps are also available.

Uses

1. For fixation of eyeball while making incision of cornea. The eyeball may be fixed at the limbus or at medial rectus muscle. It also maintains support to eyeball
2. For fixing the eyeball while passing scleral sutures
3. For packing an eviscerated or enucleated globe
4. For doing test in squint cases.

Cystitome (Capsulotomy Knife) (Fig. 9.26F)

Specifications

This is a small needle with triangular blade at the end.

Uses

1. For cutting the anterior capsule of lens in extracapsular lens extraction
2. Capsuloiridectomy after cataract
3. Needling operation.

De-Wecker's Scissors (Fig. 9.26G)

Specifications

These are fine scissors with small blades at the end oriented at an angle to the handle.

The blades are kept apart by spring action.

Uses

For cutting iris during iridectomy. The forceps are held radially to the iris and the iris is cut with single snip.

Iris Repositor (Fig. 9.26H)

Specification

It is a flat malleable blade with blunt edges and tip.

Use

To reposit the iris after iridectomy.

Desmarre's Eyelid Retractor (Fig. 9.26I)

Specifications

It has a spatulated retracting end which is bent over itself. It does not cause any damage to eye globe during retraction with spatulated end.

Uses

1. In ptosis surgery for retracting the lid.
2. It is used for double eversion of eyelid for foreign body removal
3. Used for examination of eyes in children
4. Used for examination of eyes with severe blepherospasm or extensive edema of eyelids
5. Used for fornix irrigation in cases of chemical and blast injuries.

Broad Needle (Fig. 9.26J)

Specifications

It is an oblong shaped blade with cutting edges at both sides and sharp point.

Uses

Curette linear evacuation in operation of congenital or traumatic cataract.
It may be used for paracentesis of eyes.

Iris Forceps (Fig. 9.26K)

Specifications

There are tiny forceps with fine limbs. This forceps have one into two teeth on inner side of their limbs so that when the limbs are closed, teeth cannot be felt.

Uses

1. For catching the iris tissue in iridectomy required, during cataract surgery, glaucoma surgery or optical iridectomy surgery.
2. For repairing iris tears.

Bowman's Heat Cautery (Fig. 9.26L)

Specifications

This instrument consists of a rounded ball having blunt spike. Ball tends to retain heat for a long time and cauterization done by touching the spike to bleeders. Made up of heat retaining alloy.

Uses

To heat, to cauterize the bleeders and small prolapse of iris.

Enucleation Spoon with Optic Nerve Guard (Fig. 9.26M)

Specifications

It is a curved spoon like instrument. The spooned blade has got a central cleavage to arrest the optic nerve.

Use

It is used for enucleation of the eye ball, in cases of painful blind eye.

Enucleation Scissors (Fig. 9.26N)

Specifications

It is a very small curved type of scissors, curvature is slightly upward.

Use

Used to cut the optic nerve along with its sheaths in enucleation of the eye.

Undine (Fig. 9.26O)

Specifications

It is retort shaped container with long narrow beak curved at the base. It is a glass preparation. There is an inlet to pour the solution and hole at the narrow blunt tip as outlet to irrigate. Plastic undine also is available.

Uses

To irrigate the conjunctival sac with medicated solution or normal saline during acute conjunctivitis or to wash out the eyes in other condition.

Strabismus Hook (Fig. 9.26P)

Specifications

It is a small instrument with flat hook and knobbed tip.

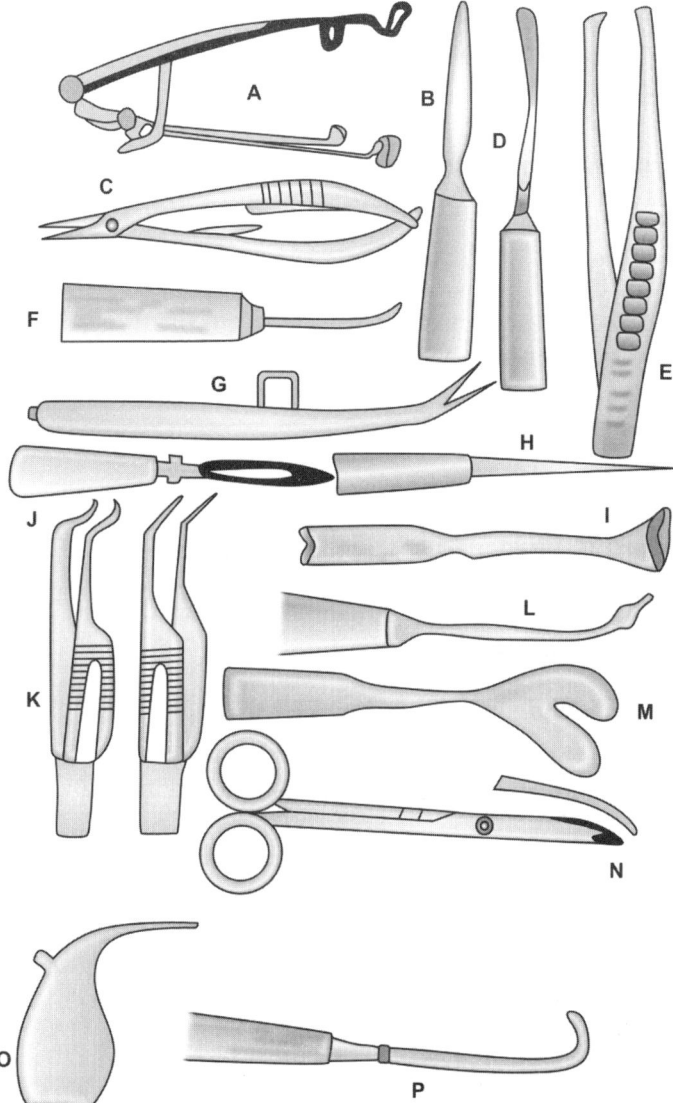

Figs 9.26A to P: Ophthalmic instruments: (A) Lang's universal eye speculum. (B) von Graefe's cataract knife. (C) Straight needle holder. (D) Curette. (E) Fixation forceps. (F) Cystitome (capsulotomy knife). (G) De-wecker's scissors. (H) Iris repositor. (I) Desmarre's eye lid retractor. (J) Broad needles. (K) Iris forceps. (L) Bowman's heat cautery. (M) Enucleation spoon with optic nerve guard. (N) Enucleation scissors. (O) Undine. (P) Strabismus hook

Uses

Used for holding and pulling on the extraocular muscles during squint and retinal detachment surgery.

ORTHOPEDIC INSTRUMENT (FIGS 9.27A TO J)

Mallet (Fig. 9.27A)

Specifications

It is a metal heavy instrument included in the orthopaedic set, named as hammer or mallet. It is also made up of Bakelite or wood, having a strong handle with a large stout and heavy head.

Uses

1. To strike on a chisel or gauge for removing bone chips
2. Used to drive in guide wires and nails in cases of internal fixation.

Chisel (Fig. 9.27B)

Specifications

Chisel is a heavy metal instrument with head, shaft and cutting edge. Head is made rounded and flat for striking with a mallet over it.

The handle is grooved to have good hold.

The cutting edge is bevelled only on one side which allows removal of sleeves of bone. It may be fully made up of metal or have bakelite handle.

Uses

1. It is used to remove sleeves of bone, e.g. bone grafting, especially for taking bone graft from the iliac crest.
2. Used for sequestrectomy, in cases of chronic osteomyelitis.
3. To remove benign growth from bones which is capped with cartilage.

Osteotome (Fig. 9.27C)

Specifications

It is just like a chisel except the cutting edge is bevelled on both sides to allow through and through cutting of bone. The handle of osteotome may be made up of metal or bakelite.

Uses

Used to cut a bone in various lengths in osteomyelitis—osteotomy. This operation is usually done to correct the length and direction of a mechanical axis of malunited or deformed bones for better mechanical advantage and for correcting congenital deformity of hip, osteoarthritis and limb disparities in the length of limbs.

Amputation Saw (Fig. 9.27D)

Specifications

This is a metal instrument named as bone saw, it may have a fixed or detachable type of blade.

Uses

It is used to cut bone with a regular surface in case of amputation required in gangrene, crush injuries of the bone, etc.

Gigli's Wire Saw (Fig. 9.27E)

Specifications

It consists of two to four strong flexible metal wires braided close together for strength and efficiency. It is about 35 to 50 cm in length. The braided wires presents rough surface like a saw, to cut sharply through the hard bone. The ends of the wire is looped at either end to be hooked into the handle by which the surgeon works with the wire saw.

Uses

1. Used for cutting the skull between trephine holes in order to reflect an osteoplastic flap in burrhole operation

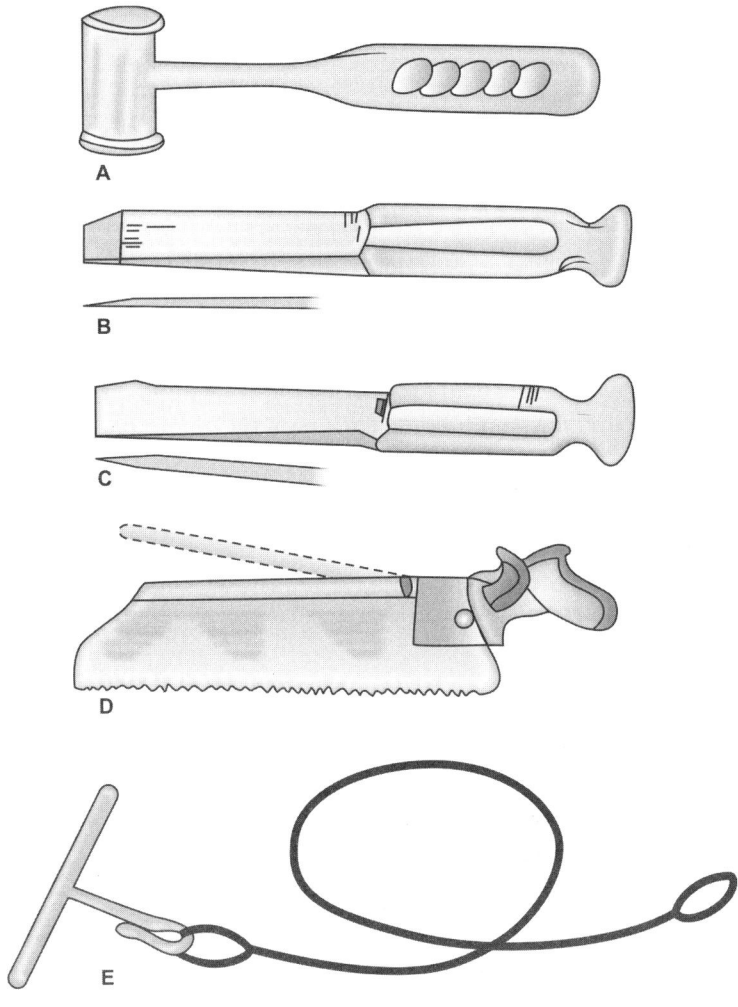

Figs 9.27A to E: Orthopedic instruments: (A) Mallet. (B) Chisel. (C) Osteotome. (D) Amputation saw. (E) Giglis wire saw

2. Used in sawing the bone lying in a deep cavity surrounded by important structures
3. Used for McMuray's osteotomy
4. Also used in pubiotomy in cases of contracted pelvis.

Bone Cutter (Fig. 9.27F)
Specifications
It is a strong heavy metal instrument with sharp blades to cut the bone.
Handles are strong and rough provided with lever arrangement for mechanical advantage.

Uses
1. It is used to cut long bones like metacarpals, metatarsals and phalanges in cases of gangrene or crush injuries
2. It can be used for cutting bony spurs.

Bone Nibbler (Fig. 9.27G)
Specifications
It is a strong metal instrument with cupped blades. The blades have sharp edges, available in various sizes. Cupped end of the blades in blunt, may be straight or angled to the handles of the instrument. The handles have a single or double action.

Uses
1. Used to nibble away small pieces of bone in various surgery of extremities and spine to smoothen the surface of the bone as in laminectomy, excision of exostosis, anterior-lateral decompression, etc.
2. To make pieces of bone for biopsy.

Charnley's Periosteal Elevator (Fig. 9.27H)
Specifications
It is a long metal instrument with a curved blade bevelled at its tip, also named as bone lever. Handle is long.

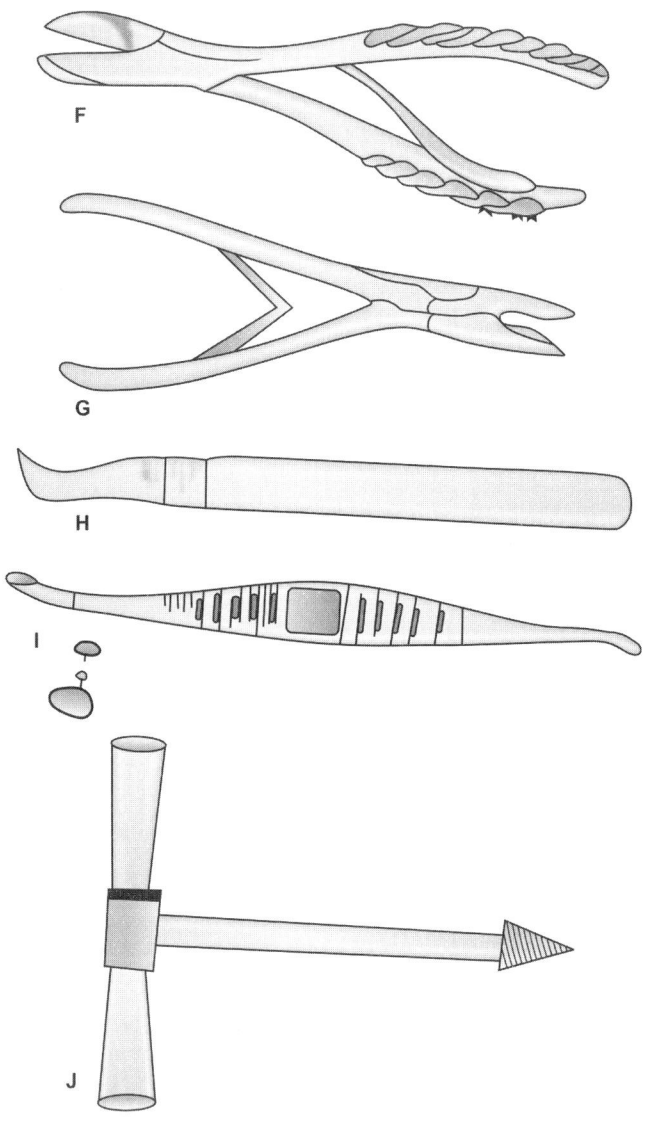

Figs 9.27F to J: Orthopedic instruments: (F) Bone cutter. (G) Bone nibbler. (H) Charnley's periosteal elevator. (I) Volkmann's scoop, and (J) Moore femoral head extractor

Uses

To lift and retract the separated periosteum, usually used to remove periosteum before removing bone for grafting.

Volkmann's Scoop (Fig. 9.27I)

Specifications

It is a long metal instrument with scooped ends, i.e. each of the ends has got cavity with sharp edges, which allows easy curettage.

Uses

1. Used for curetting bony cavities such as abscess formed due to chronic osteomyelitis
2. To curette chronic ulcers and sinuses in the bone
3. To curette out the lining of cyst in the bone
4. It can be used to pour drug in to a cavity for dressing purposes.

Moore Femoral Head Extractor (Fig. 9.27J)

Specifications

It is a heavy metal instrument with a handle, shaft and round serrated and slightly sharp head.

Uses

Used for extracting the head of the femur from the acetabulum in cases of intracapsular fracture at the neck of the femur.

UROLOGICAL INSTRUMENTS (FIGS 9.28A TO H)

Morris Kidney Retractor (Fig. 9.28A)

Specifications

It is a heavy metal instrument almost like a single blade abdominal retractor. The difference is that there is an acute bent at the junction of handle and shaft.

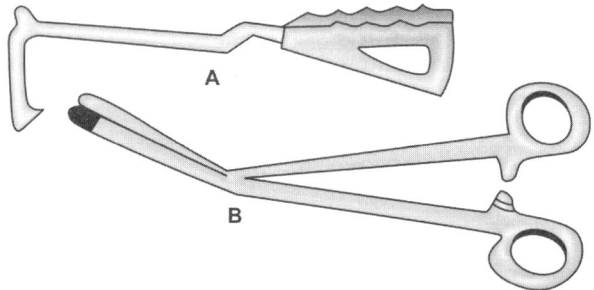

Figs 9.28A and B: Urological instruments: (A) Morris kidney retractor. (B) Renal pedicle clamp

Use

To retract tissues even at deeper level during kidney operations.

Renal Pedicle Clamp (Fig. 9.28B)

Specifications

It is a heavy metal instrument like long artery forceps but stronger than artery forceps for holding pedicles. There is a bent at 60° at the junction of shaft and blades. The bent is upwards for conveniently holding the pedicles in the depth. Catch lock is provided near the handles.

Uses

1. To clamp the pedicles in the depth
2. To hold the ligaments of uterus while doing hysterectomy.

Wheel Houses Perineal Staff (Fig. 9.28C)

Specifications

It is a rod like structure of metal instrument grooved on the stem. It is available in wooden preparation also.

Use

It is used as a guide for knife in lithotomy which is directed through the groove on the stem.

Thompson Walker's Suprapubic Cystolithotomy Forceps (Fig. 9.28D)

Specifications

It is a metal forceps like, long instrument with small blades. The blades are cupped and have a rough surface. There is no locking mechanism in this instrument so that any damage to the surrounding tissues are avoided and also any accidental crushing of the stone is prevented.

Use

It is used for holding and taking out the calculi during operation for bladder stones.

Urethral Dilators (Fig. 9.28E)

Specifications

Also called bougies. There are two types. Listen type and clutten type. It is a long slender instrument with long shaft and a blunt tip. Shaft is near its tip. There is a small circular handle which shows numbers to detect the size of the dilators. The sizes mentioned are 5/8, 7/10, 11/14, etc. Here smaller number indicates diameter of the tip and large number indicates diameter of base of dilator.

Uses

1. For dilating the urethral strictures
2. For dilating normal urethra prior of cystoscopy. Usually a normal adult urethra accommodates 11/14 sized dilator.

Bladder Sound (Fig. 9.28F)

Specifications

It is an outdated instrument used previously before the introduction of radiography and ultrasonography. It has a handle, rod like long shaft ending with a slightly bent and blunt up.

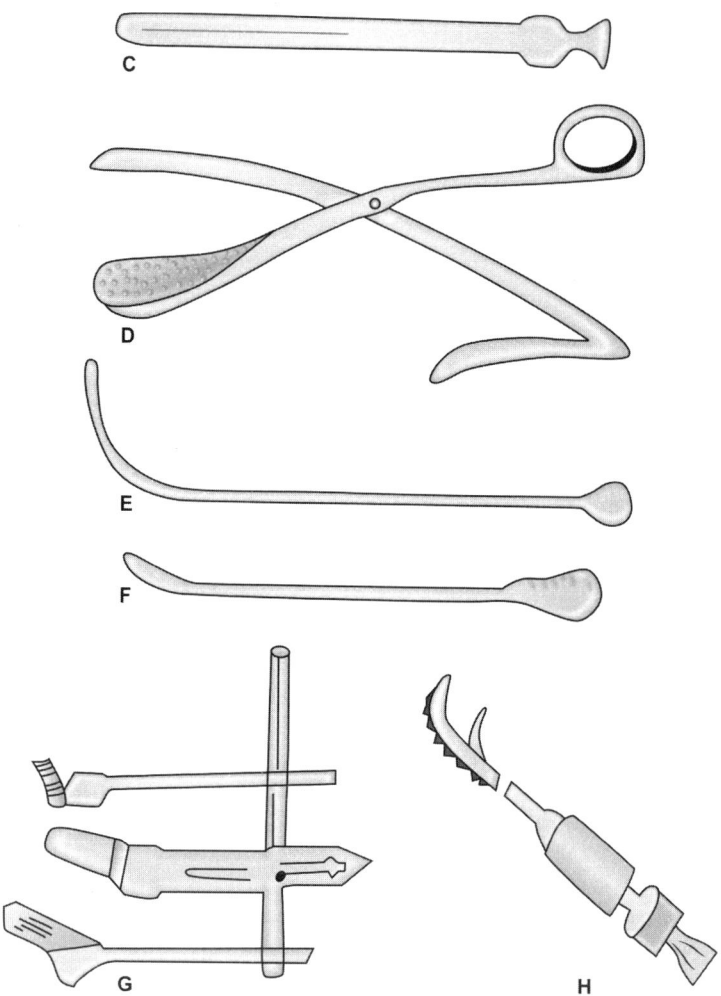

Figs 9.28C to H: Urological instruments: (C) Wheel house's perineal staff. (D) Thompson Walker's suprapubic cystolithotomy forceps. (E) Metal bougie (urethral dilator). (F) Bladder sound. (G) Thompson Walker's bladder retractor, and (H) Lithotrite

Uses

Used for exploring the interior of the bladder to detect the presence of stones by sounding.

Thomson Walker's Bladder Retractor (Fig. 9.28G)

Specifications

It is a metal instrument with three blades joined by another metal shaft in which middle adjustable for the required retraction while in use. Middle blade is detachable also.

Use

To retract the lower abdominal wall while doing suprapubic operation.

Lithotrite (Fig. 9.28H)

Specifications

It is a special instrument designed with a handle, rod like serrated body with detachable blade of two wings slightly at the tip. It is introduced into the bladder to crush the calculi in bladder.

INSTRUMENTS AIDING ANESTHESIA (FIGS 9.29A TO E)

Laryngoscope McIndoe's Curved Blade Laryngoscope (Fig. 9.29A)

Specifications

It is a metal instrument consists of a battery containing handle with a blade attached to it by hinge. A small electric bulb is situated half way along the top surface of the blade which is lit by moving blade 90° to the handle activating a switch at a hinge. The blade is 'z' shaped, in cross section to allow the tongue to be pushed to the opposite side of the mouth. The blade is curved in McIndoe's type of laryngoscope and straight in Magilli's type of laryngoscope. For children straight blade type is more useful.

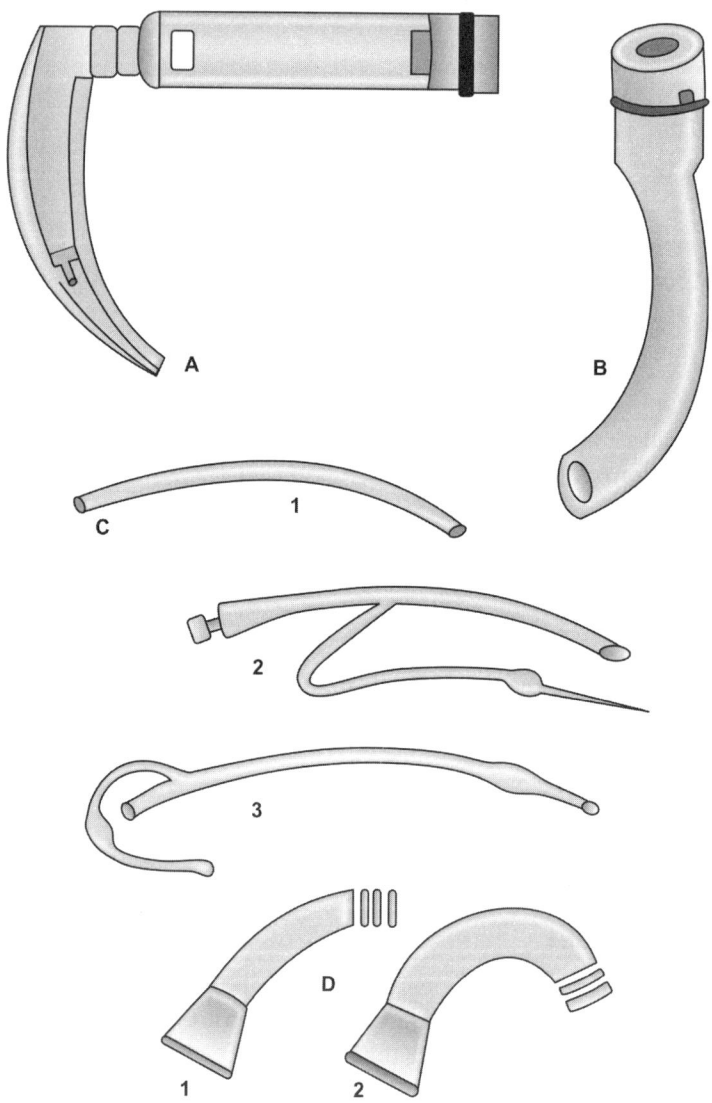

Figs 9.29A to D: Instruments aiding anesthesia: (A) Laryngoscope (Mackintosh's curved blade laryngoscope). (B) Gudel's oropharyngeal airway. (C) Endotracheal tubes; (1) Plain, (2) Cuffed red rubber, and (3) Protex cuffed tube. (D) Endotracheal connections: (1) Oral, and (2) Nasal

Blades are of various sizes and detachable and interchangeable. Usually adult size is used for all patients except very small children.

The laryngoscope blade consists of the spatula the flange and the tip.

Use

It is used for direct examination of larynx and for intubation during anaesthesia or assisted ventilation.

Guedel's Oropharyngeal Airway (Fig. 9.29B)

Specifications

Oropharyngeal airway is made up of hard rubber or plastic which is the widely used airway nowadays. It is a hollow plastic or rubber tube bend at the shaft according to the curve of the oropharynx with full opening of the tube at the tip. At the proximal end there is a round metal connection joining the plastic tube to provide easy handling during introduction and prevent collapse of the tube between the teeth.

Uses

1. Used to prevent biting and obstruction of endotracheal tube
2. To prevent obstruction of natural air passage by relaxed tongue and soft pharyngeal tissue during induction and recovery from anesthesia
3. It also facilitates suctioning of pharyngeal secretions through the hole of the airway.

Endotracheal Tube (Fig. 9.29C)

Specifications

Endotracheal tubes are made up of red rubber (Magill variety) or other synthetic materials like pvc and polyethylene. Endotracheal tubes may be cuffed or non-cuffed.

Different types of endotracheal tubes are available according to the internal diameter of tubes in millimeters.

Uses

Endotracheal tubes are required to administer anesthesia where face mask cannot be used; it is possible to give positive pressure ventilation with endotracheal tubes, particularly with cuffed tubes, as they make an airtight connection with trachea.

Endotracheal Connectors (Fig. 9.29D)

Specifications

Endotracheal connector is designed as to permit rapid disconnection and reconnection of endotracheal tubes. Few connectors have provision for suction. The connectors for nasal tubes have special angulation. They can be autoclaved.

Uses

The endotracheal connectors are used to join endotracheal tube to the mouth or adaptor between breathing attachment and endotracheal tube.

Nasopharyngeal Airways (Fig. 9.29E)

Specifications

They are made up of hard rubber or plastic designed with metal connection at the proximal end. Length and inner diameter varies according to the size. The distal end is completely opened.

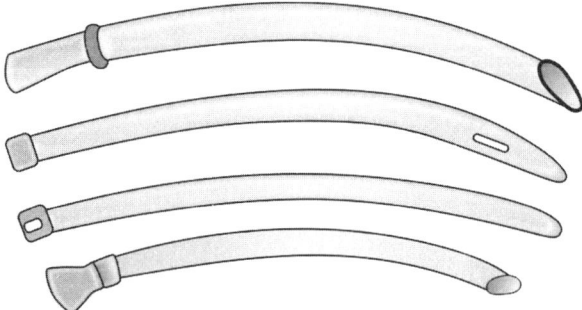

Fig. 9.29E: Instruments adding anesthesia: Nasopharyngeal airways

Preferably oval shape with blunt end, which will prevent damage to the tissue while introducing.

Use

This hollow nasopharyngeal tube is inserted into a nostril and directed along the floor of the nose to the nasopharynx to prevent the tongue from blocking off air passage in an unconscious patient.

10 Anesthesia

Anesthesia is a complex highly developed science. The anesthetic nurse or the technician work with the anesthetist and help him. So the anesthetic nurse, assistant or technician must familiarise themselves with the basic principles of anesthetic apparatus and the use of anesthetic drugs in the particular theater in which they work.

GENERAL LAYOUT OF THE ANESTHETIC ROOM

Anesthetic room should be of the same hygienic construction as the theater and sterilising room. If there are more than one anesthetic room in a multiple theater suite, equipment should not be interchanged between rooms and to avoid this it is important to ensure that adequate replacements are available.

All anesthetic rooms should contain dust-proof cupboards, having an adequate number of wide shelves with an impervious surface. Equipment stored in these cupboards is laid neatly on the shelves, labeled and in order. All items must be clearly visible and always kept in the same place. Items such as laryngoscopes should be duplicated as they are known to fail to crucial moments. It is better to have another place to store for general replacements. Various sizes of endotracheal tubes, etc. may be keep separate by storing them complete with their connectors, in individual paper bags.

Separate locked cupboards should be reserved for scheduled "DDA" (dangerous drugs administered) and the keys carried by the anesthetic nurse or theater sister on duty. These cupboards may also contain the register used for recording dangerous drugs administered to the patient in theater. It is the legal obligation of the anesthetist to enter all use made of dangerous drugs, the name of the patient and quantity used. Drugs for immediate use may be stored in a locked drawer fitted to the anesthetic machine.

A small wash basin with elbow operated mixing taps and requisites for scrubbing up should be provided in the anesthetic room. This basin should be positioned away from areas in which sterile trolleys are being used.

An adequate suction machine or pipe line suction device must be available, together with a suction tube and selection of suction nozzles and catheters with connectors of proper size.

A dispenser should be provided containing a selection of disposable sterile syringes in sizes ranging from 2 ml to 20 ml, hypodermic and intravenous needles. In addition to general diffused lighting, a small maneuverable spotlight, wall or ceiling mounted is useful during intravenous procedures.

Two trolleys about 45 cm (18 inches) square are necessary for the exclusive use of the anesthetist for transfusions and local anesthetic techniques.

At least two transfusion stands should be available, a Martin transfusion pump to enable rapid transfusion of blood should be fitted to one or ideally to each of the stands, to supplement the pumping device of plastic recipient sets.

Essential equipment always ready for use should include a *sphygmomanometer*, stethoscopes, tracheostomy set, cardiac arrest set and transfusion sets. Access to a defibrillator and monitoring apparatus is essential. All movable equipment is positioned suitably for anesthetist's convenience.

TYPES OF ANESTHESIA

The main types of anesthesia are:
1. General anesthesia
2. Local or regional anesthesia
3. Spinal and epidural anesthesia

General Anesthesia

It is induced by inhalation of gases or the vapor of volatile liquids which vaporise readily at normal room temperatures. These include:

Nitrous Oxide

Stored in cylinders in a liquid form, under pressure, often referred to simply as 'gas'. Nitrous oxide is a weak agent of which high concentration (50-60%) are used in conjuction with other anesthetics and oxygen.

Cyclopropane

A potent gas stored in cylinders in a liquid form and used only in low concentrations (15%). It is flammable and explosive and therefore, must not be used in the presence of cautery or diathermy.

Ether

A volatile liquid which has a wide margin of safety in use although prolonged inhalation can cause postoperative vomiting and depression, has an unpleasant, irritant smell, is inflammable and explosive when mixed with O_2.

Halothane (Fluothane)

A volatile liquid which is neither inflammable nor explosive. It's characteristics include lack of irritation of the respiratory tract; effectiveness in low concentration, rapid recovery after administration, absence of side effects such as vomiting.

Methoxyfluorane (Penthrane)

Similar to halothane but vaporises less readily; induction and recovery are slower has analgesic properties in low concentration.

Trichloroethylene (Trilene)

A blue colored liquid with a relatively slow rate of vaporization. Trilene has a predominantly analgesic effect and is used to supplement other gaseous anesthetics. Used alone as a 0.5 percent mixture in air; it can be administered in small amounts in child birth to relieve pain without loss of consciousness, cannot be used in a closed circuit in the presence of sodalime, which is incompatible with Trilene.

General Anesthesia Induced by the IV Administration of Drugs

Such as the short acting barbiturates. The most commonly used in this class are thiopentone sodium (Pentothal), methohexitone sodium (Brietal) and nonbarbiturates such as propanidid (Epontol) a very short acting agent, ketamine hydrochloride (ketalar) and Althesin, a steroid anesthetic agent. Epontol is very suitable for use in accident and dental departments. Other drugs, although they may not be anesthetics in themselves, are often used in combination with those listed above.

Local Anesthesia

It is induced by surface application, local infiltration of regional nerve block and epidural or subdural spinal injection of drugs such as procaine (Novocaine), lignocaine, (xylocaine), amethocaine (decicaine), prilocaine (citanest), bupivacaine (marcaine) and cinchocaine (nupercaine). Cocaine is used for surface application only, e.g. ophthalmic surgery.

Induced Hypothermia

It is a state of lowered body temperature produced by physical cooling of patients who are under the effect of a general anesthetic, and the so-called lytic cocktail of which the most important element is chlorpromazine (Largactil, Megaphen).

Neuroleptanalgesia

It is a state of indifference and insensitivity to pain induced by the intravenous administration of a potent analgesic drug combined with a transquilliser, e.g. phenoperidine (operidine) or fentanyl (sublimaze) combined with a butyrophenone transquilliser such as droperiodol (Droleptan) or haloperidol.

The patient is easily rousable with a normal blood pressure and when awakened remains quite. He is in a state of apathy and mental detachment in which he is mildly sedated and uncaring about his surroundings.

Preparation for Anesthesia

1. The gas cylinders and soda lime canister, a box or container for carbon dioxide absorbent etc on the anesthetic machine are checked by an experienced anesthetic nurse or technician and reserves of these, together with bottles of halothane (Fluothane), trilene and ether are kept nearby.
2. The anesthetic nurse also sets out instruments and apparatus required by the anesthetist. She or he prepares trolleys and trays when necessary for open ether, intravenous anesthesia, endotracheal intubation, and local regional or spinal analgesia.

The Anesthetic Machines

There are many varieties of anesthetic machines. Although most operating theaters are now supplied with piped gases, each machine must be fitted with oxygen and nitrous oxide cylinders for emergency use in case of failure of piped gas supplies.

Anesthetic gas cylinders are colored in accordance with a British standard's institute code. Oxygen cylinders are painted black with a white top and O_2 printed in black, nitrous oxide are blue with N_2O printed in black, cyclopropane are orange, with C_3H_6 printed in black and CO_2 are painted grey with CO_2 also in black.

Regulators are attached to each cylinder to reduce the high pressure gases, thereby making delivery easily adjustable through individual rotameters which control the amount of gases flowing into the machine and to the patient. There is a cylinder content gauge either for each cylinder or fitted between two cylinders of the same gas.

Before connecting a new cylinder, after the protective cap has been removed, the valve should be opened momentarily to expel any dust which may have lodged in the valve seating. Modern anesthetic machines incorporate cylinder which have valves of the 'pin index type' which cannot be connected to the incorrect regulator. The fiber washer between the cylinder and cylinder yoke or regulator yoke must be changed regularly as it becomes worn.

The cylinder valve must be centred correctly with the cylinder yoke or regulator yoke and the holding screw turned carefully into its location on the back of the valve using hand pressure only. A leak at this point when the valve is opened usually indicates a worn or absent washer or the gas cylinder being connected or the wrong pin index yoke.

Important

On no account must any grease be used on cylinders regulators or connections, for the friction produced by the gas may ignite the grease and cause an explosion.

Varieties of an Anesthetic Machines (Figs 10.1 to 10.4)

There are many different types of anesthetic machines manufactured. Three main types are:
1. A semi-closed circuit Boyle's type to which can be added a closed circuit
2. Similar to 1 but incorporating a ventilator
3. A self-contained CO_2 absorption circle (closed) circuit.

These machines are designed to use pipeline gas supplies; plus reserve cylinders. For pipeline gas supplies the machine is connected to the pipeline outlet by flexible rubber hoses incorporating self sealing sehrader connectors. In addition the machines are generally fitted with two nitrous oxide cylinder, two oxygen cylinders and one CO_2 cylinder. There may also be provision for cyclopropane (C_3H_6) but the gas cylinder should be removed from the machine when not in use to eliminate the explosion hazard due to its explosive properties.

The high-pressure gases passes through regulators to the rotameters and then into a common supply tube either direct to the patient or are diverted through the halothane trilene or ether vaporiser and then to the reservoir bag. From this bag the gases are carried via the corrugated rubber tube, angle piece and face

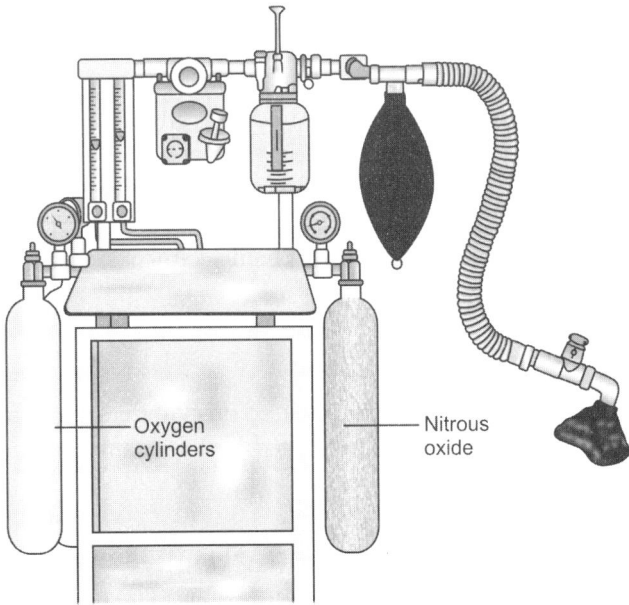

Fig. 10.1: Basic Boyle's anesthetic machine

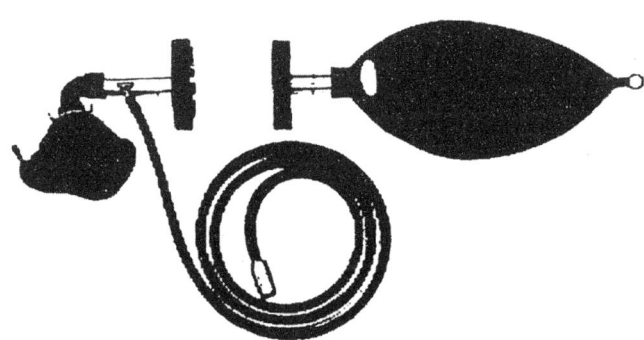

Fig. 10.2: Waters 'to and fro' carbon dioxide absorption canister

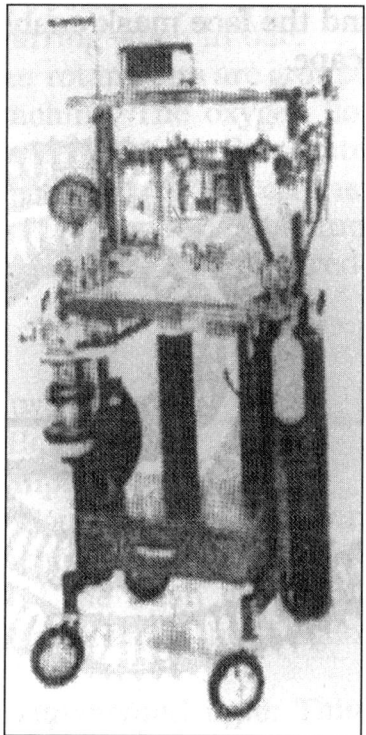

Fig. 10.3: Anesthetic machine (Boyle international specification model)

mask or endotracheal tube to the patient. Adjustment of an expiratory valve situated between the corrugated tube and the face mask enables expiration and excess gases to escape.

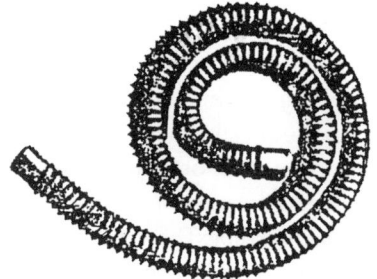

Fig. 10.4: Corrugated breathing tube

Regulator or reducing valves on anesthetic machine are usually of the Adam's or Endurance type and they reduce the high gas pressure to the minimum. This enables easy delivery of the gases through individual high pressure rubber tubes or soldered metal tubes to the control flowmeters. A separate regulator is used for each gas cylinder. An aneroid gauge attached to the regulator indicates the pressure of the cylinder contents.

Rotameters

A rotameter (flowmeter) is an accurately, made conical glass tube containing a 'float' or bobin which rises and rotates as the flow of gas increases. The flow meter must be set perfectly vertical, otherwise the float will not spin round. Rotameters are individually calibrated according to the type and quantity of gas used. With the exception of cyclopropane, the flow of gases is controlled by a fine adjustment needle valve on the rotameter. Cyclopropane is generally controlled directly from the cylinder by a special key, circular being the safest to avoid accidental jarring when in use.

The three or four rotameters are grouped together, feeding gases into the machine. The oxygen flow meter is always placed at the extreme left of the flow meter bank followed by the cyclopropanes, CO_2 and N_2O on the extreme right. An oxygen by pass lever supplies emergency oxygen when an increased flow of pure oxygen is required.

Vaporizers

Vaporizers are of two types:
A. The standard Boyle type
B. The thermo-compensated type
A. *The standard Boyle type:* This incorporates a valve or slotted drum which allows the anesthetist to divert a portion or all of the fresh gases above the surface or through the volatile anesthetic agent before passing to the patient.
B. *The thermo-compensated type:* This type, e.g. fluotec has replaced the standard vaporizer for the modern tendency is to use vaporizers producing known concentrations. With these

vaporizers known percentages of halothane can be added to the fresh gases of any standard continuous flow anesthetic apparatus. The concentration of halothane is controlled by the restrictions of the temperature sensitive thermostat and the control channel. The restrictions of the thermostat alters according to the operating temperatures.

Pin safety system: This consists essentially of noninterchangeable bottle units which fit the combined filler and drain of the vaporizer.

The reservoir bag made of thin anti-static rubber is generally of a 1 gal: (4.5 liters) capacity. The anesthetic gases enter this bag via a drum valve, which is generally a permanently open 'T' junction. This bag should be tested regularly for leaks by inflating and submerging in water. There is a tendency for cracks to appear in the folds. After prolonged use, the reservoir bag is removed from its mount and inverted to drain off condensed moisture vapor, prior to cleaning and sterilization.

The corrugated tube made of anti-static rubber and having a wide bore is joined to the machines at one end and the angle piece at the other by slightly conical metal or hard rubber unions. The union at the angle piece incorporates an expiratory valve. The tube must be checked regularly for punctures as there's a tendency for deterioration to occur in the corrugations. After use it should be stretched and suspended straight for a period, to release condensed moisture which is often lodged in the corrugations and then sterilized at least at the end of a list if not after each operation.

The expiratory valve: On modern apparatus, it is usually of the Heidbrink. This is a spring-loaded valve upon which tension may be adjusted to create a slight resistance against the patients expirations. When closed circuit is used the valve is completely closed and it is necessary to cut the gas flow down to basic oxygen requirements.

The metal angle piece connects to the face mask, made from anti-static rubber manufactured in a modified funnel shape which, when applied to the patient's face with the facial contours forming an airtight fit. The basic types are (a) those having a solid or moulded lip of suitable design and (b) those having an inflatable cushion.

The trilene inter-lock unit is mounted in the circuit between the trilene vaporizer and the reservoir bag. This drum valve is so designed that the trilene vaporizer control can not be moved from the 'off' position unless the drug is set at open circuit. The inter-lock device also incorporates an emergency O_2 level which enables the administration of a plentiful supply of O_2 to the patient if the need arises.

An antistatic rubber harness: May be used by the anesthetist to maintain the face mask in position.

An endotracheal tube and connection may be attached directly to an expiratory valve and the corrugated tube by substituting a magill catheter connection for the angle piece and face mask. In this case the corrugated tubes and expiratory valve are supported carefully, to avoid pulling on the endotracheal tube after insertion, which can be achieved by using adhesive strapping.

An airway may be used in the patients mouth to prevent the tongue from falling back, and also prevent teeth clenching an endotracheal tube.

The CO_2 Absorption Circle Closed Circuit Added to the Basic Boyle's Machine

In the circle apparatus, two corrugated tubes are used, one for the delivery of gases to the patient through a one-way inspiration valve, and another through which the expiratory gases are directed into the re-breathing bag-via another one way expiration valve. The patient's expirations from the reservoir bag pass through the soda lime canister and a selected proportion of CO_2 is removed. The expirations then mix with fresh gases from the rotameters, which may have been passed through the vaporizer. This gas mixture is directed through the inspiration valve and along the corrugated tube back to the patient, thereby completing the circuit.

Modern sodalime preparations such as calona (BOC) or Durasorb (MIE) contain a colored indicator, which retains it's color so long as the sodalime remains active. After 4-6 hours use, Durasorb changes from a pink to a cream color and should be replaced. Calona indicates exhaustion by a change from green to brown. Many machines are now fitted with transparent absorber canisters which permit the color of the sodalime to be easily observed.

Anesthetic Machine with Ventilator

Ventilators can be utilized along with anesthetic machine (Basic Boyle's apparatus). An example is *Blease Northwick Park Anesthetic trolley*. This machine has the characteristics of a Boyles apparatus, but incorporates a variable frequency, variable phase, time cycled pressure or volume limited ventilator. The ventilator is operated entirely by the gas delivered through the anesthetic unit to the patient. A sensitive manometer, recording both positive and negative pressure, is fitted to the unit. This machine incorporates a closed circle circuit CO_2 absorption units.

The Marrett Circle Circuit Machine

This is a compact apparatus which easily transportable when a suitable cylinder stand is incorporated.

The machine consists of two main parts—the head and cylinder stand or table. The head is supplied with gases in the usual manner from cylinders and regulators fitted to a circular stand or anesthetic table. Four moderately high-pressure rubber or soldered metal tubes convey the anesthetic gases from the regulators to the bank of four rotameters on the anesthetic head. The head has two vaporizers one for ether or halothane and one for trilene together with a sodalime canister, all of which are controlled by three separate circular knobs which actuate complicated drum valves.

The ether vaporizer uses special copper baffle plates, 4-6 in number which conduct the heat from the rest of the apparatus and surrounding atmosphere, thereby aiding the vaporization of the ether or halothane. The trilene vaporizer has a smaller bottle than the ether, and consists of a single perforated tube terminating below the level of the liquid.

An interlocking device is provided to prevent trilene being used when the sodalime has been turned on and vice versa.

A circle or closed circuit has many advantages including the conservance of expensive anesthetic vapors or gases such as cyclopropane and halothane; the very accurate control of anesthetic agents and degree of anesthesia using minimal anesthetic, the conservance of body moisture and heat.

Ventilators

Ventilators are used to achieve controlled respiration during anesthesia or following traumatic condition such as head injuries. This may be accomplished simply by rhythmically squeezing the anesthetic reservoir bag or by mechanical ventilators.

Basically ventilators could be divided into 3 main groups.
1. *Flow generators:* A fixed volume of gases is delivered into the lungs. A wide variation in the pressure reached at the end of inspiration may be observed on the manometer gauge. Fibrosed and stiff or congested lungs, airway obstruction including excessive secretion, foreign body, bronchospasm, etc. all will require high pressure valves. When the pressure reach at a certain level, usually 40-70 cm of water, a safety valve blows off a proportion of the given volume.
2. *Pressure generators:* With these the ventilators produces a selected pressure within the limits of time imposed by the respiratory rate. The amount of gases required for this pressure depends upon the compliance of the lungs and chest.
3. *Ventilators providing a choice of volume of pressure:* Some ventilators are electrically driven (with a manual control for emergency), others convert a continuous flow of oxygen or compressed air from a cylinder into an intermittent flow to the patient.

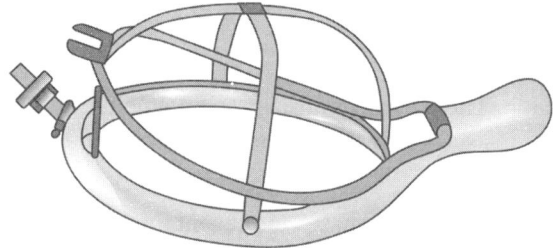

Fig. 10.5: Open ether: Schinamel Busch mask

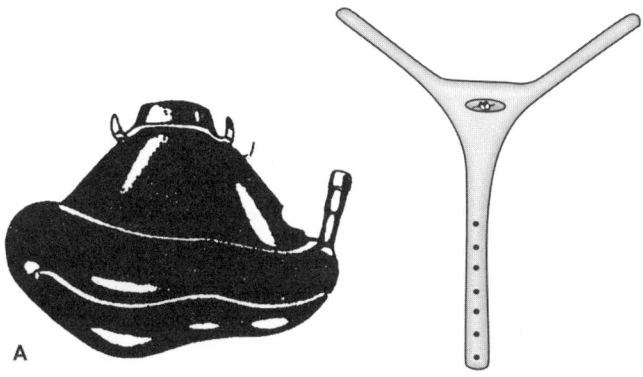

Figs 10.6A and B: (A) A face mask, and (B) Harness

Even with the advent of the newest and complicated anesthetic techniques, the administration of open ether is still used occasionally and might well be valuable in the event of a major disaster.

Induction of anesthesia is accomplished by the patient breathing through a gauze pad on to which is dropped a quantity of ether. Initially, ethyl chloride is commonly used to induce unconsciousness, because it is less unpleasant to breathe than the ether vapor (Figs 10.5 to 10.7). The thickness of gauze shall be adequate to prevent the drops of ether from falling on the patients face. As the outer edges of the gauze can become moistened with either during a long period of anesthesia, it is preferable to cut this gauze pad to the mask shape.

A piece of gamagee measuring about 23.5 cm by 35.6 cm and having a central slit exposing the nose and mouth, is placed to protect the face. A similar piece is placed over the mask and ether dropped through the slit on to the underlying gauze.

In order to minimise the risk of burns from liquid anesthetic, petroleum jelly can the applied to the lips and sterile castor oil droops for the eyes after the ether has been administered. These should always be available when open ether is being administered.

178 Operating Room Technique and Anesthesia

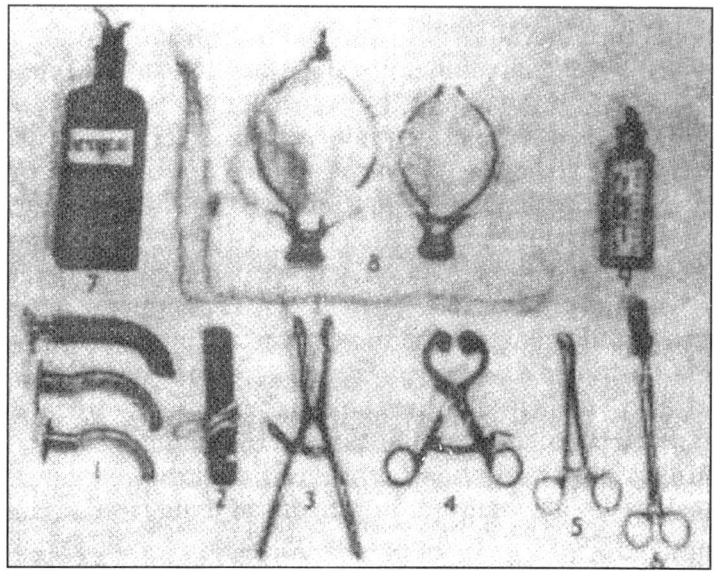

Fig. 10.7: Open ether requirements: (1) Airways (2) Boxwood wedge (3) Mouth gag (4) Tongue forceps. (5) Tongue clip. (6) Pharyngeal swab-holding forceps. (7) Ether bottle. (8) Open inhalers (adult and child), and (9) Ethyl chloride

Intravenous Anesthesia (Fig. 10.8)

A selection of intravenous anesthetic agents, relaxants stimulants, and antidotes should be clearly labeled and available for the anesthetist.

The intravenous barbiturates in common use are thiopentone sodium (Pentothal) 2.5%, methohexitone sodium (Brietal) 1% and the hypnotic propanidid (Epontol) 5% and Ketamine hydrochloride. A 2.5% solution is prepared by dissolving 0.5 g in 20 ml of sterile pyrogen-free distilled water respectively. Phenoperidine, pethidine and pentazocine are used extensively. Pethidine is often diluted to 1% solution containing 10 mg/ml.

Relaxants in common use include the "competitive blocker" muscle relaxants such as curare (Tubarine), gallamine triethiodide (Flaxedil), pancuronium bromide (Pavulon) and depolarising muscle relaxants such as suxamethonium (Scoline).

Stimulants in common use include nikethamide (coramine) aminophylline, methedrine, methoxamine, metaraminol, noradrenalin and

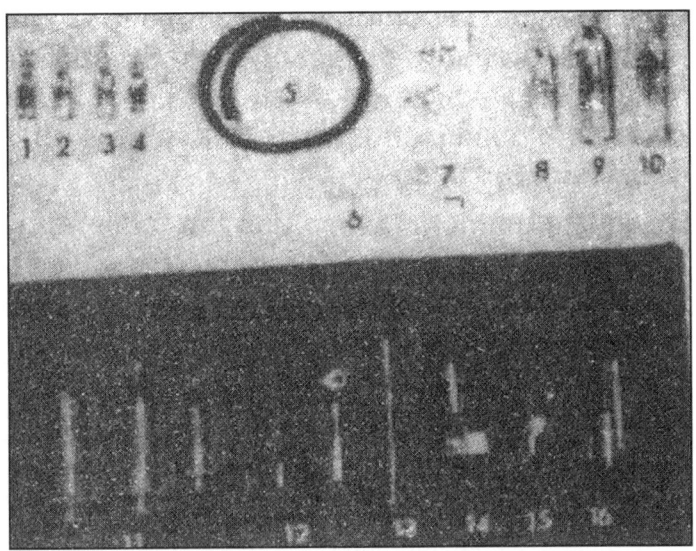

Fig. 10.8: Requirements for the intravenous induction of anesthesia

1. Succinylcholine (Scoline)
2. Curare (Tubarine)
3. Pethidine (DDA) Dangerous Drug Administration
4. Atropine
5. Rubber tubing for tourniquet
6. File
7. Spirit-swabs
8. Propanidid
9. Water for injection
10. Thiopentone sodium (Pentothal)
11. Disposable syringes (Pentothal) 20 ml, 10 ml, 2 ml
12. Hypodermic needles No. 20, 12 and 1 with needles case
13. Disposable filling cannula
14. Disposable gordh needle
15. Mitechell needle, tourniquet
16. Disposable needles (Plextrocan)

adrenaline. Antidotes commonly needed include atropine, prostigmine, nalorphine, etc.

It is the anesthetist's responsibility to prepare these solutions, but if the anesthetic nurse is permitted to do so, she should check the preparation with a second person and show the anesthetist the ampoules from which the injection has been prepared.

The sizes of needles used vary with individual choice. For continuous or intermittent intravenous injections, either the syringe and needle are left in position so that small quantities may be injected as required; or a special needle such as butterfly is left in the vein. Continuous intravenous anesthesia can be maintained by using a very weak intravenous solution, which is administrated via a saline transfusion or small quantities of the drug can be injected into the rubber transfusion, as required.

When preparing different solutions at a time, it is necessary to label syringes to aid identification.

Endotracheal and Endobronchial Intubation

Apparatus for passing an endothracheal tube must be ready before the commencement of any anesthetic induction (Fig. 10.9). Laryngoscopes used when introducing an endotracheal tube include the Magill straight blade and the anatomical shaped blade Mackintosh types. There are 4 basic types of endotracheal tubes, the nasal type and the oral type, both cuffed and non-cuffed.

The Endotracheal Tube is Used

1. When in the opinion of the anesthetist, the airway is liable to be obstructed
2. For operation in which it is necessary because of surgical technique, e.g. head and chest operations
3. For upper abdominal operations and artificial ventilation
4. When the towelling and position of the patient prevents the anesthetist gaining easy access to the patient's head, and thus guaranteeing a free airway, e.g. craniotomies
5. To prevent the inhalation of blood or vomit, e.g. emergencies
6. In the treatment of cardiac arrest.

Anesthesia **181**

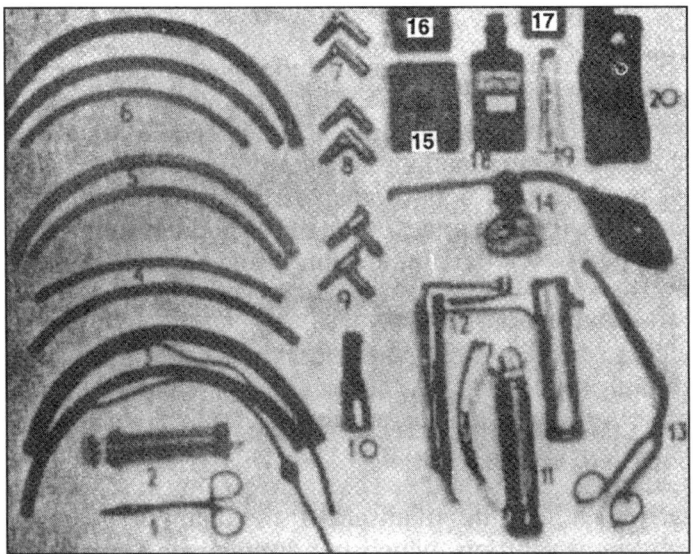

Fig. 10.9: Requirements of endotracheal intubation

1. Artery forceps
2. 10 ml syringe
3. Endotracheal tubes, cuffed (Magill)
4. Endotracheal tubes, nasal (Magill)
5. Endotracheal tubes, oral, plastic (Magill)
6. Endotracheal tubes, oral, rubber (Magill)
7. Endotracheal tubes, connections (Row botham)
8. Endotracheal tube connections (cobb, plain type)
9. Endotracheal tube connections (cobb with suction access)
10. Endotracheal catheter mount (Magill) (Mackintosh)
11. Laryngoscope (Mackintosh)
12. Laryngoscope (Magill)
13. Endotracheal tube forceps
14. Atomizer for topical anesthesia
15. Catheter mount clip
16. Gauze roll for pharyngeal pack
17. Anesthetic swabs
18. Local anesthetic for topical application
19. Tube lubricant
20. Endotracheal head harness (Hudson)

The anesthetist generally is likely to use an endotracheal tube which has a terminal cuff which when, inflated with air, impinges upon the tracheal mucosa, thereby sealing the lungs from the upper respiratory passages to prevent the inhalation of blood or vomit. The amount of air used for inflation may vary from 2 ml and 10 ml of air. Nasal tube size may vary from 3 mm-12 mm according to the age of the patient.

The experienced anesthetic nurse or technician will learn to select the sizes and type of endotracheal tubes required. When cuffed tubes are to be used, they must always be tested by inflating the cuff before handling to the anesthetist. All the apparatus should be laid out in the order required, giving special attention to the provision of correct size tube connections and laryngoscopes in good working order. The electric lamp on the laryngoscope must illuminate brightly. A second laryngoscope must always be available in case of lamp failure during use. A tube of lubricant is usually required and this may be combined with a local anesthetic such as 2% lignocaine. A suction machine with long suction catheters is prepared, together with a small bowl of clean water for rinsing the catheters.

The endobroncheal tube is in effect of an extended cuffed endotracheal tube of smaller dimensions, which is passed into the left or right bronchus. Endobronchial tubes have an inflatable cuff, to isolate the intubated lung. The anesthetist will require a bronchoscope of suitable type, in addition to laryngoscope and may also need a long bronchial spray with a surface anesthetic, e.g. lignocaine.

All endotracheal and endobronchial tubes must be cleaned thoroughly with a brush and warm antibacterial detergent solution after use. Those having inflatable cuffs are checked before being stored away, care being taken to avoid water entering the cuff. The tubes are sterilized after use.

After use, laryngoscope blades should be dismantled from the battery handle, cleaned and sterilized by autoclaving.

2. Local or Regional Anesthesia (Fig. 10.10)

This may range from a simple injection for infiltrating a small area to an extensive nerve block.

A 10 ml or 20 ml syringe is adequate for minor procedure.

A fine hypodermic needle of size 18 or 20 will be required for the initial 'weal', followed by a longer one of wider bone. A selection of needles should be available ranging from 2-4 inch in length and 20-26 BWG in gauge.

Most commonly using anesthetic agents are lignocaine (xylocaine) bupivacaine (Marcaine) and procaine. A 1.5 or 2% lignocaine is used for the initial infiltration. Where larger quantity is necessary, the strength of solution is reduced to 1% or 0.5% and the amount injected limited to the maximum dose of the agent. (e.g. the max dose of plain lignocaine (xylocaine) in a normal healthy adults is 13-15 ml of a 1.5% solution, 23 ml of a 1% solution or 46 ml of a 0.5% solution). Dosage must be reduced in the ill and elderly.

In order to produce vasoconstriction, and thereby lesson capillary hemorrhage, adrenaline may be added in the proportion of 1 in 400,000 to 1 in 100,000 according to the total amount of solution being injected. A 1 in 400,000 solution may be prepared by adding 1 ml of 1 in 10,00 adrenaline to 399 ml of local anesthetic agent. A 1 in 100,000 solution may be prepared by adding 1 ml of 1 in 1000 adrenaline to 99 ml of anesthetic agent. A 1 in 100,000 addition of adrenaline also prolongs the action of the local anesthetic by delaying absorption up to six hours, and thereby increases the safety margin for larger doses. If the anesthetic nurse is permitted to prepare injections, she should always check the preparation with the anesthetist, retaining all containers for anesthetist inspection.

Following operation, when a local anesthetic has been administered, great care must be taken to avoid injury to areas which may remain analgesic for several hours. This applies especially to the use of hot water bottles and electric pads or blankets as postoperative measure.

The topical application of anesthetic agents such as cocaine to the eye and lignocaine, etc. to the mucosa of the mouth, pharynx of respiratory tract requires special aftercare. The eyes must always

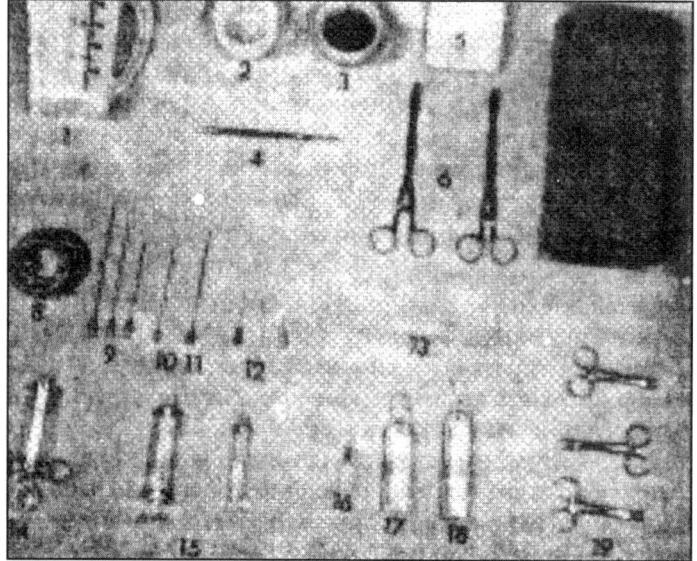

Fig. 10.10: Requirements for local or regional anesthesia

1. 0.5 liter measuring jug
2. Skin antiseptic
3. Bonney's blue for marking infiltrated area
4. Skin pen and nib
5. Green swabs
6. Sponge holding forceps
7. Sterile towels
8. Self-filling attachment
9. Locking needles
10. Bracheal plexus needles
11. Filling needles
12. Hypodermic needles
13. File
14. Syringes (Labet)
15. Syringes (10 ml and 20 ml)
16. Adrenaline
17. Lignocaine
18. Distilled water
19. Towel clips

be covered for several hours. Even with a minor operation, a patient who has had an application of local anesthetic to the mucosa of the respiratory tract is not permitted to eat or drink for at least 4 hours following operation and can cough effectively, as the resultant paralysis of the soft palate and epiglottis would allow foreign matter to enter the trachea. Watch also for possible reactions to the local anesthetic including convulsions. If there's the slightest doubt or history of previous sensitivity a small test dose doubt should be given first.

3. Spinal and Epidural Anesthesia (Fig. 10.11)

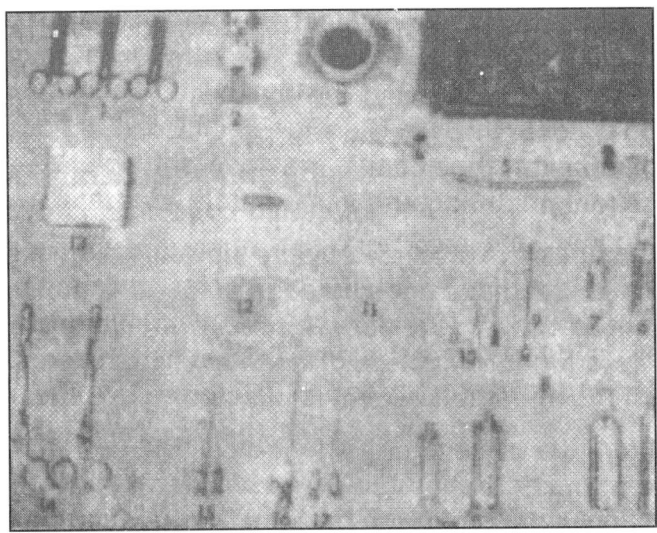

Fig. 10.11: Requirements for spinal and epidural anesthesia

1. Towel clips
2. Sterile CSF specimen bottle
3. Aqueous skin antiseptic
4. Sterile towels
5. Spinal manometer and connecting tube
6. Bupivacaine (Marcaine) with 1 in 200,000 adrenaline
7. Cinchocaine (Heavy nupercaine)
8. File
9. Filling needle
10a. Hypodermic needles size 20, 12 and 1
10b. Hypodermic needles size 20, 12 and 1
11. Three-way tap
12. Epidural plastic cannula
13. Green swabs
14. Sponge holding forceps Rampley (2)
15. Epidural needles
16. Spinal needle
17. Spinal needles
18. Syringes 2 ml and 10 ml
19. Sterile distilled water
20. Lignocaine 1.5% (xylocaine)

These requirements should always be autoclaved before use in a special spinal packet.

Spinal anesthesia is produced by making a spinal intrathecal injection of a heavy or light solution of anesthetic agent such as cinchocaine, lignocaine and bupivacaine. In spinal anesthetic the drug mixes with the cerebrospinal fluid and bathes a portion of the spinal cord and nerve roots, thereby rendering part of the body analgesic as well as paralysing the muscles. The extent of its desired action is determined by the anesthetist and depends upon the volume of solution, the specific gravity of the solution and the position of the patient during and immediately after injection.

Epidural analgesia is produced by the slow injection of a larger volume of local anesthetic agent into the epidural space between the ligamentum flavum and the dura. A special needle or cannula is used to facilitate the introduction of an indwelling nylon catheter through which the anesthetic agent is injected.

For injection, the patient may either be sitting up with his legs over the side of the operation table and head and shoulders bent forwards or lying on the side with his legs drawn up, the head and shoulders being bent towards his knees.

Storage of Equipment for Anesthesia

Rubber should be stored at temperature below 21°C. No lubricant based on liquid paraffin should be used; it ruins rubber.

Drugs should also be stored at relatively low temperature. The reserve stock and those particularly sensitive to heat such as scoline and heparin should be kept in a refrigerator.

The Patient

When a patient comes to the theater, with a certain amount of apprehension, the manner in which he is treated may seriously affect the induction of anesthesia and his subsequent recovery. He should be made to think that he is the center of attention and that all possible skill is being used for his welfare.

The patient should always be accompanied to the theater by a ward nurse, and if possible this nurse should remain with him until the induction of anesthesia is complete. The psychological effect of this is very good, for the patient feels reassured by the presence of ward nurse who is often the person responsible for his nursing after the operation.

The patient must be accompanied by X-rays, case notes, signed consent for anesthetic and operation, pathological reports and drug sheet and any other relevant information which will be of use to the surgeon or the anesthetist. The ward nurse should know the preparation which the patient has had, the time at which food or drink was last taken, the type and amount of preoperative drugs administered and the time at which they were given. She is responsible for seeing that any dentures have been removed, and must know whether the patient has passed urine or has been catheterized and the time and amount passed, together with any abnormalities detected in routine ward tests.

The patient is brought to operating department on his bed or trolley and he is transferred to a theater trolley before entering the sterile zone. The patient is anesthetised on the trolley or may be transferred on the underlying canvas stretcher to the operation table in the anesthetic room.

A patient must never be left alone in the anesthetic room or theater for he may be confused following preoperative drugs and this may lead to accidental personal injury, like fall polley.

Identification of patient, his correct operation and correct site is of paramount importance. This procedure starts in the ward where some identifications of the patient's name and case number must be attached to him before he is transferred to theater. In unconscious patient operation site should be marked with an indelible marker indicating the correct side or digit or identification can either be in the form of a bracelet or details written on the patient by means of a skin pen.

On arrival at the theater the patient's identification is checked against the case notes and operation list. If conscious, he is further asked his name. The anesthetic and operation consent form must also be checked. The surgeon should see the patient before anesthesia is induced and confirm it is the correct patient, operation and site. The nurse should see that the patient is kept as quiet as possible and should not encourage conversation unless it is obvious that the patient feels more relaxed doing so.

During induction the nurse stands by in case the patient becomes restless, but if he does, she must not attempt to wrestle with him but must apply gentle restraint, with one arm across the legs just above the knee, using the other arm to prevent any wild flinging about if the patient's arms.

For intravenous injection, the selected arm is extended towards the anesthetist and either a quick-release tourniquet applied to the upper arm or the nurse constricts the venous return by encircling the upper arm with her hands. The patient clenches his fist to make the veins prominent, and after the anesthetist has aspirated blood into the syringe, the compression of the upper arm veins is released at the anesthetist's request. The nurse stands at the head end of the trolley or operation table to support the patient's jaw when relaxation is complete. The anesthetist will then apply pressure over the area of injection, which is continued by the nurse when the inhalation anesthetic is commenced.

The basis of keeping an airway clear is supporting the jaw and extending the head. The nurse should place her fingers behind the angle of the jaw on each side, lifting it slightly forwards. This will pull upon the muscle attachments of the tongue, preventing it from the falling backwards and thereby maintaining an unobstructed channel between the mouth and larynx.

An unobstructed airway is indicated by quiet respirations, as noisy breathing is obstructed breathing. The position of the head

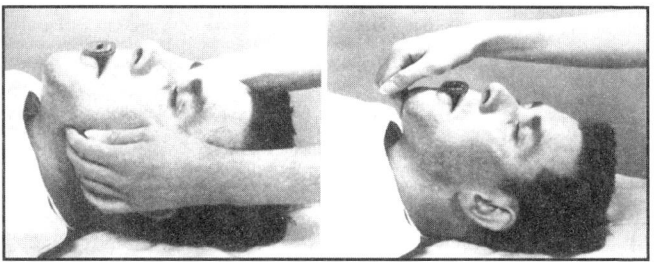

Fig. 10.12: Supporting the jaw of an unconscious patient

or lower jaw may require adjustment to achieve this object (Fig. 10.12). So the nurse should use her hands, sense of hearing and observe the patient's color and respiration.

As the patient loses consciousness, following the IV injection of a barbiturates and relaxant especially in emergency situations it is possible for regurgitation of stomach contents to occur before the anesthetist has inserted the endotracheal tube. The nurse may be required to perform the sellick maneuver as soon as unconsciousness intervenes.

The sellick maneuver consists of temporary occlusion of the upper end of the esophagus by backward pressure of the cricoid cartilage against the bodies of cervical vertebrae. This prevents regurgitation of oesophageal or stomach contents during induction of anesthesia, and also prevents gastric distension from positive pressure ventilation administered by facemask (or mouth to mouth resuscitation).

As soon as unconsciousness intervenes, firm pressure can be applied without obstructing the airway and this is maintained until the endotracheal tube has been inserted and the cuff inflated.

The nurse should not speak during the initial stages of anaesthesia, as it is possible for the patient's hearing to become acute. She should not begin to remove the bandages or covers until the patient is complete unconscious.

The anesthetic nurse will hand instruments to the anesthetist as required and will try to anticipate his requirements.

Anesthetic nurse may be assigned to observe the condition of patient during anesthesia and keep a record of the patient's pulse, respiration, blood pressure, color etc. She will adjust the rate of flow of transfusion, indicated by the anaesthetist and replace transfusion solutions under his directions.

Guedal Describes Four Stages of Anesthesia

The first stage is one analgesia when peripheral sensation is lost, but the nervous system is under control. In the first stage of induction there are frequently swallowing movements, followed by regular respiration and analgesia.

The second stage is one of excitement, with movements of the limbs followed by tonic spasms of the muscles, dilated pupils and moving eyeballs. Quite often this stage is very short and almost absent, especially when anaesthetising the deeply sedated patient.

The third stage is the stage of surgical anesthesia which may range from moderate to deep according to the type of operation.

The fourth stage which is respiratory and cardiac arrest.

If the patient collapses on the operation table with acute cardiocirculatory arrest his recovery may well depend upon prompt action by all theater staff. Without treatment, irreversible damage may occur in 3 minutes and a lasting recovery of the brain and thus the whole body is impossible after 8 minutes.

CARDIOCIRCULATORY ARREST

If this has occurred immediate steps are taken to restore adequate ventilation and circulation. The anesthetist will be required to keep a record of time from the first warming. He tilts the operationable head downwards, stops the anesthetic, ensures that the airway is clear and administers oxygen under pressure. He may later pass an endotracheal tube if one is not already inserted.

At the same time, the surgeon commences external cardiac massage. It can be done by rhythmic external manual compression of the sternum which in turn compress the heart between it and the spine; forcing out blood into the aorta and allows it to fill with blood. Patient should be kept on a rigid surface similar to the operation table. The compression on the lower half of the sternum must be by the heels of the hands, on top of the other, aided by the weight of the body.

Depression of the sternum should be at least 3-4 cm with each stroke, with a frequency of between 70 and 90 strokes/minute. This should produce a palpable radial pulse with a blood pressure of 80-100 mm Hg. Rhythmic compression of the sternum does not produce effective ventilation. This must be accomplished either by manual compression of the anesthetic machine bag or attachment of the endotracheal tube to a ventilator.

Immediately cardiac massage has been started, the circulating nurse or anesthetic nurse fetches the cardiac resuscitation set which comprises various drugs, transfusion fluids and equipment, syringes and needles, electrical defibrillator and if possible an electrocardiograph monitor, which should be connected to the patient.

When ventricular systole is responsible for the arrest of circulation, external massage may re-establish normal rhythm. If there is no response, intracardiac injections may be tried. The most generally used is adrenaline 1 in 10,000 dosage 3-5 ml. Intracardiac or adrenaline 1 in 10,000, 1 ml/minute intravenously. This is for myocardial stimulation.

Calcium chloride, 10% may be given intracardiac or intravenously in a dosage up to 10 ml. This increases tone in flabby heart. These measures may provoke ventricular fibrillation which can then be treated with a DC counter shock administered by the defibrillator. The shock should be given starting at 300 J/2 to 4 millisecond. If a defibrillator is unavailable, ventricular fibrillation can sometimes be treated by intravenous procaine amide 1 g propranolol (Inderal) 5 mg given slowly.

If the period of arrest exceeds 2 minutes or if cardiac massage has been carried out for longer than 15 minutes, the patient should have 200/500 ml of 4.2% sodium bicarbonate intravenously to prevent acidosis. If pulmonary edema is suspected or if the volume of intravenous fluid given has exceeded 1500 ml, a diuretic may be given. If normal consciousness does not return fairly quickly, there may be cerebral edema which may be treated by intravenous 50% sucrose.

General Outline of Procedure for Cardiocirculatory Arrest

1. Arrested heart
2. External massage, controlled pulmonary ventilation
3. No beat, adrenaline given or attempt with DC shocks
4. Fibrillation of the heart
5. DC defibrillator applied using large moistened, firmly attached electrodes with a surface area of at least 10 cm and supplying in adults 300-400 JDC over 2-4 millisecond
   All staff take *hands off patient* to avoid a personal electric shock

6. Beat recommences
7. Intravenous transfusion of 200/500 ml of 4.2% sodium bicarbonate plus possibly noradrenaline to maintain blood pressure
8. Endotracheal tube passed at earliest opportunity, artificial ventilation continued until normal respiration recommence
9. If external massage unsuccessful, direct massage by a thoracotomy may be considered. If the chest is opened, antibiotics should be given.

CARDIAC-RESPIRATORY ARREST TROLLEY

Contents

Top of Trolley

Airways: Sizes 4-00	Elastoplast 75 cm
Laryngoscopes: Adult blade	IV cut down set
Child blade	IV fluid
Pen torch	Disposable giving set
Tongue depressor Intracatheter	
Mouth gag	2 IV needles
Magills forceps	Stethoscope
Tongue forceps	Receiver with suction
20 ml syringe	catheters.

Middle Shelf

Bronchoscopy Tray	Connections (3)
Tracheostomy tray (sterile) (with suture materials)	Ambu bag to endotracheal tube
	Cyclator to tracheotomy
	Cyclator to endotracheal
Hemorrhage arrest tray (sterile)	Gauze and lubricant
	Strapping: 12 mm

Bottom Shelf
Defibrillator
Electrode jelly

Suction unit
Rubber gloves
Battery unit
Cyclator pump

Scissors
2 way resuscitation tubes (6)
Sizes from 00/000 to 3/4
Labels
Biro
Emergency drugs
Gord H Needle (sterile)
Sterile intracardiac needle

Left Side Trolley
Extension lead
Oxygen cylinder
Ambu Resuscitator

Drugs on Trolley
Calcium chloride 10% 10 ml
Atropine sulphate 0.6 mgm
Aminophylline: 250 mgm

Right Side of Trolley

Drip stand
Oxygen cyclator
Cylator bracket

Attached to back of Trolley
Cardiac Arrest Board

Lid of Trolley (with Night Light)
Endotracheal Tubes (8)
Sizes from 9.5 to 5.5 with connections (sterile)

Suxamethonium (Scoline) 100 mgm
Nikethamide 2 ml
Digoxin 0.5 mgm

Adrenaline 1/10,000

Lorfan 1 mgm
Prostigmine 2.5 mgm

Methyl amphetamine, 30 mgm

Spencer wells artery forceps		Methoxamine 20 mgm
		Hydrocortisone sol 100 mgm
Book for recording used items		Noradrenaline 100 mgm
Sphygmomanometer		Procaine amide 100 mgm in 1 cm^3
3 files		Procaine hyd. 10% 20 ml
		Lignocaine 1% 10 ml
Needles	4 No. 15	Vandid 5% A
	4 No. 1	Propanolol 5 mgm in 5 ml
Syringes	1 ml: 3	Inj. Isoprenaline 5 mgm
	2 ml: 3	Inj. Aramine 2 mgm
	5 ml: 3	Lasix 20 mgm in 2 ml
	10 ml: 3	
Drug box (with lid)		NaHCO$_3$ BP 8.4% or 4.2% (Sodium bicarbonate BP)

When the operation is completed, the anesthetist will give instruction to the nurse accompanying the patient back to the ward. When the patient is fit to transfer, the anesthetist will say to do so.

A good airway must be maintained. If there is a possibility to vomit, he should be placed on his side with the underlying limb flexed and the shoulders supported.

The patient is transferred carefully to the ward trolley with minimal movement and covered with blankets before leaving the theater suite. He should be handled very gently, not only to avoid injury to the operation area, but a sudden rapid movement of the unconscious patient can cause cardiac arrest.

A tray containing mouth gag, tongue forceps, wooden wedge, small towel and kidney tray should be carried with the patient during transit between the theater and ward. These instruments must remain by the bed until the patient has recovered consciousness.

An airway or endotracheal tube left in position by the anesthetist postoperatively *should not be removed* until the patient attempts to reject it. Attempts at rejection by the patient reveal that his swallowing reflex has returned and that unless there's any clinical contraindication, the tube may be removed.

If oxygen has to be administered postoperatively to an unconscious patient, it should be given by means of a suitable catheter, mask or oxygen tent. If an endotracheal tube is in position, oxygen may be given via a catheter passed into the lumen of the tube for a few inches. The oxygen flow in this latter case should not be above 3 liters/minute.

BIBLIOGRAPHY

1. Raymond J., Brigdon S.R.N. Operation Room Tech.

Index

A

Abscess incision (opening an abscess) 64
Absorbent materials 30
According to use 29
Adenoid curette with cage 138
Airway 174
Allis tissue forceps 107
Amputation saw 151
Amputations 65
Anesthetic machine with ventilator 175
Anesthetic machines 168
Aneurysm needle 29,110
Anorectal instruments 132
Anterior vaginal wall retractor 104
Antistatic rubber harness 174
Antrostomy 35
Appendicectomy 35
Appendicostomy 35
Arthrodesis 35
Arthroplasty 35
Arthrotomy 35
Aural speculum 115
Autoclaving 19
Auvard's weighted vaginal speculum 116

B

Balfour's self-retaining retractor 102
Bard Parker knife handle 94
BP handle and blades 94
Bladder sound 159
Boilable instruments 26
Boiling 20
Bone cutter 153
Bone grafting 66
Bone nibbler 153
Bowman's heat cautery 148
Boyle-Davis mouth gag 133,141
Broad needle 147
Bronchoscopy 35, 68

C

Cardiac-respiratory arrest trolley 192
Cardiocirculatory arrest 190, 191
Care of specimens 52
Carton-Cowell's mucous catheter 129
Cataract extraction 90
Categories of people in the operating room 3
Catgut 30
Cauterization 69
Cesarean section 35, 69
 lower segment operation 69

Charnley's periosteal elevator 155
Cheatle's forceps 112
Chevalier Jackson's direct laryngoscope 142
Chisel 150
Cholecystectomy 35, 69
Cholecystectomy or gallbladder position 15
Cholecystenterostomy 35
Cholecystotomy 35
Choledochotomy 35
Chordotomy 35
Circumcision 70
Cleft palate repair 71
CO_2 absorption circle closed circuit 174
Colostomy 35, 70
Colporrhaphy 36, 70
Corrugated tube 173
Craniotomy 36
Crocadile punch biopsy forceps 133
Curettage 36
Curette 145
Curve 28
Cusco's bivalved speculum 119
Cyclopropane 166
Cystectomy 36
Cystitome (capsulotomy knife) 145
Cystolithotomy forceps 157
Cystoscopy 36, 71
Czerny's retractor 103

D

De-Wecker's scissors 146
Deaver's retractor 101
Denis Browne tonsil holding forceps 135
Dental extraction 72
Desmarre's eyelid retractor 146
Diathermy 36
Dilatation and curettage 72
Disinfection by chemicals 21
Dissecting forceps 96
Double hook retractor 100
Doyen's retractor 100
Drew-Smythe catheter 125
Dry heat 20

E

Ear, nose and throat instruments 133
Ectomy 34
Ectopic gestation 36
Embolectomy 36
Enamel and other metal ware 33
Endotracheal and endobronchial intubation 180
Endotracheal connectors 162
Endotracheal tube 162, 174
Ent operations 86
Enucleation of eye 90
Enucleation scissors 148
Enucleation spoon with optic nerve guard 148
Epididymectomy 36

Episiotomy 37
Episiotomy scissors 124
Esophagoscopy 39, 80
Ether 166
Eve's tonsillar snare 135
Examination for patency of the fallopian tubes 84
Excision jaw 73
Expiratory valve 173
Eye dressings 24
Eye operations 90

F

Fistula director 132
Fixation forceps 145
Floss silk 32
Flow generators 176
Flushing curette 122
Frer's septal knife 134

G

Gastrectomy 37, 74
Gastroenterostomy 37, 74
Gastroscopy 37
Gastrostomy 37
General anesthesia 166
General anesthesia induced by the IV administration 167
General functions of operating room nurses 4
General layout of the anesthetic room 164
General set of instruments 63
Gigli's wire saw 151
Gloves 22

Gloving 12
Gowning 12
Green: armytage forceps 125
Guedal describes four stages of anesthesia 189
Guedel's oropharyngeal airway 161
Gum elastic and plastic materials 23
Gynecological and obstetric instruments 120

H

Halothane (fluothane) 166
Hegar's cervical dilator 120
Hemorrhoidectomy 75
Hemostats (artery forceps) 98
Herniotomy 37, 75
Hodge's pessary 128
Hydrocele 37, 75
Hymenectomy 37
Hysterectomy 37

I

Ileostomy 37
Induced hypothermia 167
Insertion of radium 76
Instruments 26
Instruments aiding anesthesia 159
Interlocking device 175
Internal urethrotomy 84
Intestinal resection 76
Intranasal ethmoidectomy 88
Intravenous anesthesia 178
Iridectomy 37
Iris forceps 147

J

Jackson's tracheostomy tube 141
Jejunostomy 37
Joll's thyroid retractor 103

K

Kelly's deep retractor 101
Killiani's self-retaining nasal speculum 116
Kocher's forceps 99

L

Lacks spatula 139
Laminaria tent 129
Laminaria tent introducing forceps 129
Laminectomy 37, 77
Langenbeck's retractor 101
Lang's universal eye speculum 115, 144
Laparotomy 38, 74
Laparotomy position 14
Laryngeal forceps 134
Laryngectomy 38
Laryngofissure 38
Laryngoscope Mcindoe's curved blade laryngoscope 161
Laryngoscopy 38
Laryngostomy 38
Leucotomy 38
Ligatures 64
Ligatures and sutures 30
Linen thread 31
Lister's sinus forceps 110
Litholapaxy or lithotrity 38

Lithotomy position 14
Lithotrite 159
Living sutures 30
Lobectomy 38
Local anesthesia 167
Local or regional anesthesia 183
Long bladed nasal speculum 115
Luc's forceps 134
Lumbar ganglionectomy 78

M

Major abdominal incisions 113
Mallet 150
Marrett circle circuit machine 175
Mastectomy 38
Mastoid gouge 139
Mastoid retractor 141
Mastoidectomy 86
Meniscectomy 38
Metal 32
Metal angle piece 173
Methods of suturing 114
Methoxyfluorane (penthrane) 166
Moore femoral head extractor 155
More details about needles 28
Morris kidney retractor 156
Moynihan's tetra clip 93
Myoma hook 128
Myomectomy 38
Myringotome 139
Myringotomy 39

N

Nail brushes 33
Names of general instruments 91

Nasopharyngeal airways 163
Needle holder 108
Needles 86
Nephrectomy 39, 79
Nephrectomy or kidney position 14
Nephropexy 39
Nephrostomy 39
Nephrotomy 39
Neuroleptanalgesia 167
Nitrous oxide 166
Non-absorbent materials 31
Nonboilable instruments 27
Nylon thread 31

O

Obstetrical forceps 131
Oophorectomy 39, 80
Operating room—physical set up 1
Operating table 13
Operations 66
    on the breast 66
    on the genitourinary tract 71
    on uterus and fallopian tubes 76
Ophthalmic instruments 144
Orchidectomy 39
Orrhaphy 34
Orthopedic instrument 150
Oscopy 34
Osteotome 151
Osteotomy 39
Ostomy 34
Other bone operations 67
Otomy 34

Overiostomy 39
Overiotomy 39
Ovum forceps 122

P

Pan-hysterectomy 37
Partial gastrectomy 74
Payr's gastric crushing clamp 106
Perineorrhaphy 39, 80
Peritonsillar abscess drainage forceps 135
Pharyngotomy 39
Phrenic avulsion 39
Pile holding forceps 133
Pin safety system 173
Pneumonectomy 40
Pneumothorax 40
Polypectomy 88
Polypus forceps 126
Position for bronchoscopy and esophagoscopy 17
Position for cerebellar operations and high lamine 16
Position for operations in the neck 16
Positions for operations on the breast and axilla 15
Postpartum sterilization 86
Premedication room 53
Preparation 8
    anesthesia 168
    anesthetic table 8
    ether soap 11
    sterilization 21
    theater and equipment 9
Pressure generators 176

Probe 112
Proctoscope 133
Proctoscopy 81
Prostatectomy 40
Pyelogram (retrograde) 40
Pyelolithotomy 40

R

Radical or Wertheim's hysterectomy 37
Rammstedt's operation 40
Rampley's sponge-holding forceps 91
Recovery room 53
Regulator or reducing valves 172
Removal of nasal polyp 88
Renal pedicle clamp 156
Reservoir bag 173
Responsibilities of the circulating nurse 49
Retractors 100
Retrograde pyelography 71
Rotameters 172
Rubber goods 21
Rubins' tubal insufflation cannula 126

S

Salpingography 85
Scissors 95
Scrubbed nurse 42
Scrubbing 10
Setting up of sterile trolley 9
Signaloc 19
Silk thread 31
Silkworm gut 31

Simpson's uterine sound 120
Sims' double ended uterine curette 121
Sims' vaginal speculum 119
Single hook retractor 100
Skin grafting 82
Small single hook retractor (tracheal hook) 142
Smith's pessary 128
Special positioning of the operating table 14
Speculums 115
Spinal and epidural anesthesia 185
Splenectomy 40
Standard Boyle type 172
Sterile water and infusion fluids 25
Sterilization 18
Sterilization by heat 18
Strabismus hook 150
Straight needle holder 144
Suction nozzle and tubing 105
Suprapubic cystostomy 82
Suprapubic prostatectomy 80
Surgical dressings and linen drapes 23
Suture needles 28, 109
Syringes and glass wares 32

T

Tarsorrhaphy 40
Team work 3
Tenaculum forceps 124
The endotracheal tube is used 180

Thermo-compensated type 172
Thickness and size 28
Thompson Walker's suprapubic 157
Thomson Walker's bladder retractor 159
Thoracectomy 40
Thoracoplasty 40
Thoracoscopy 40
Thyroidectomy 82
Tilley nasal dressing forceps 141
Tonsillar dissector and anterior pillar retractor 138
Tonsillectomy curettage of Aden 88
Total hysterectomy 37
Towel clips 92
Tracheostomy 40, 89
Tracheostomy instruments 141
Trendelenburg position 15
Trephining 41
Trichloroethylene (trilene) 166
Trilene inter-lock unit 174
Trocar and cannula 111
Trousean's tracheal dilating forceps 144
Types of anesthesia 165

U

Undine 148
Ureteric catheterization 71
Ureterolithotomy 41
Urethral dilators 157
Urethrotomy 41, 83
Urological instruments 156
Uterine packing forceps 125

V

Vacuum cups 131
Vaporizers 172
Vasectomy 85
Ventilators 176
Ventriculography 41
Ventrosuspension 41
Vesical 41
Vesicovaginal fistula 85
Volkmann's scoop 155
von Graefes cataract knife 144
Vulsellum forceps 122
Vulvectomy 41

W

Wheel houses perineal staff 157
Willett's scalp traction forceps 131